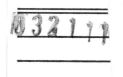

the**facts**

Tourette syndrome

➲ also available in the**facts** series

Eating disorders: the**facts**
SIXTH EDITION
Abraham

Epilepsy: the**facts**
THIRD EDITION
Appleton and Marson

Osteoarthritis: the**facts**
Arden, Arden, and Hunter

Asthma: the**facts**
Arshad and Babu

Sexually transmitted infections: the**facts**
SECOND EDITION
Barlow

Autism and Asperger syndrome: the**facts**
Baron-Cohen

Epilepsy in women: the**facts**
Betts and Clarke

Living with a long-term illness: the**facts**
Campling and Sharpe

Chronic fatigue syndrome: the**facts**
SECOND EDITION
Campling and Sharpe

Head injury: the**facts**
Daisley, Tams, and Kischka

Falls: the**facts**
Darowski

Infertility: the**facts**
Davies, Overton, and Webber

Prenatal tests: the**facts**
De Crespigny and Chervenak

Obsessive-compulsive disorder: the**facts**
THIRD EDITION
de Silva

Polycystic ovary syndrome: the**facts**
Elsheikh and Murphy

Muscular dystrophy: the**facts**
THIRD EDITION
Emery

Psoriatic arthritis: the**facts**
Gladman and Chandran

The Pill and other forms of hormonal
contraception: the**facts**
SIXTH EDITION
Guillebaud

Cystic fibrosis: the**facts**
FOURTH EDITION
Thomson and Harris

Lupus: the**facts**
SECOND EDITION
Isenberg and Manzi

Ankylosing spondylitis: the**facts**
Khan

Borderline personality disorder: the**facts**
Krawitz and Jackson

Inflammatory bowel disease: the**facts**
Langmead and Irving

Stroke: the**facts**
Lindley

Diabetes: the**facts**
Matthews et al.

Essential tremor: the**facts**
Plumb and Bain

Huntington's disease: the**facts**
SECOND EDITION
Quarrell

Panic disorder: the**facts**
SECOND EDITION
Rachman

Osteoporosis: the**facts**
Reid and Black et al.

ADHD: the**facts**
Selikowitz

Down syndrome: the**facts**
THIRD EDITION
Selikowitz

Sleep problems in children and adolescents:
the**facts**
Stores

Motor neuron disease: the**facts**
Talbot and Marsden

Thyroid disease: the**facts**
FOURTH EDITION
Vanderpump and Tunbridge

Depression: the**facts**
Wasserman

Cosmetic surgery: the**facts**
Waterhouse

Alcoholism: the**facts**
FOURTH EDITION
Manzardo et al.

the**facts**

Tourette syndrome

SECOND EDITION

MARY M. ROBERTSON

Emeritus Professor in Neuropsychiatry,
University College London.
Honorary Consultant Psychiatrist,
Department of Neurology,
St George's Hospital, London.
Visiting Professor, St George's Hospital Medical
School, London.

ANDREA E. CAVANNA

Consultant in Behavioural Neurology,
Queen Elizabeth Psychiatric Hospital,
Birmingham.
Honorary Research Fellow,
Institute of Neurology,
University College London.

OXFORD
UNIVERSITY PRESS

OXFORD

UNIVERSITY PRESS

Great Clarendon Street, Oxford OX2 6DP

Oxford University Press is a department of the University of Oxford.
It furthers the University's objective of excellence in research, scholarship,
and education by publishing worldwide in

Oxford New York

Auckland Cape Town Dar es Salaam Hong Kong Karachi
Kuala Lumpur Madrid Melbourne Mexico City Nairobi
New Delhi Shanghai Taipei Toronto

With offices in

Argentina Austria Brazil Chile Czech Republic France Greece
Guatemala Hungary Italy Japan Poland Portugal Singapore
South Korea Switzerland Thailand Turkey Ukraine Vietnam

Oxford is a registered trade mark of Oxford University Press
in the UK and in certain other countries

Published in the United States
by Oxford University Press Inc., New York

© Oxford University Press 2008

British Library Cataloguing in Publication Data

Data available

Library of Congress Cataloguing in Publication Data

Robertson, Mary M.
  Tourette syndrome / Mary M. Robertson, Andrea Cavanna.
  p. cm. -- (The facts)
  ISBN 978-0-19-929819-8
  1. Tourette syndrome.   I. Cavanna, Andrea E. II. Title.
  RC375.R63 2008
  616.8'3--dc 22

                                                            2008028857

ISBN 978-0-19-929819-8

10 9 8 7 6 5 4 3 2 1

Typeset in Plantin
by Cepha Imaging Pvt. Ltd., Bangalore, India
Printed in China through
Asia Pacific Offset

Tourette Syndrome
Association of Australia Inc.

PO Box 1173 Maroubra NSW 2035
ABN 76 104 434 459
Phone (02) 9382 3726 Fax (02) 9382 3764
email: info@tourette.org.au
website: www.tourette.org.au

TSAA is a voluntary and non-profit organization consisting of people with TS, their families, health and education professionals and other interested and concerned people.

Tourette Scotland holds events and provides information, training, advice and support for people living and working with TS. We can offer information on TS specific to Scotland, e.g. education/law.

Tourette Syndrome
Foundation of Canada

La Fondation canadienne
du syndrome de la Tourette

Established in 1976, the Tourette Syndrome Foundation of Canada is the only national, voluntary, not-for-profit organization assisting individuals affected by Tourette Syndrome and its associated disorders in Canada. It is dedicated to improving the quality of life for those with, or affected by, Tourette Syndrome through programs of education, advocacy, self-help and the promotion of research. It has as its vision that all people who have Tourette Syndrome will lead quality lives as accepted and valued members of an informed, tolerant society. www.tourette.ca

The Tourette Syndrome Foundation of Canada logo is a registered trademark of the Tourette Syndrome Foundation of Canada and used under license by Oxford University Press.

Tourettes Action (UK)
Tourettes Action welcomes the publication of the new edition, which brings people with Tourette Syndrome and their families up-to-date with the latest thinking and practice.

Tourette Syndrome Association (USA)
Founded in 1972, the Tourette Syndrome Association is the only national, voluntary health organization in the US for people with TS, and has a three-pronged mission of education, research and service. For more information about TS, call (00)1-888-4-TOURET or visit www.tsa-usa.org.

Preface to the second edition

We are delighted at the positive response that we had to the first edition of *Tourette syndrome: the facts*, which was published in 1998. However, since then the literature on Tourette syndrome (TS) has mushroomed and many new scientific discoveries have taken place. Therefore we felt that it was time for a new edition to appear, reflecting these changes.

This, and the specific feedback we have received, suggests that individuals who have TS, parents of children with TS, and others need a short summary of facts and figures about the syndrome. As before, although the book is intended primarily for a lay readership, we believe that it will be useful to teachers and educationalists, doctors, psychologists, social workers, and other allied health professionals. We are very much aware of the substantial recent research published about TS and therefore we have almost completely rewritten this second edition. Since the book is aimed at a predominantly UK readership, we have concentrated on describing the UK legislation with regard, for example, to teaching and education. This second edition has different authors; Professor Robertson has been very fortunate in recruiting Dr Andrea Cavanna who is one of the best trainees she has had the pleasure of working with and who has both the academic and writing skills to ensure that the new edition is fully up to date, relevant to current practice, and intelligible. We have found the experience of collaborating on this new edition to be both intellectually stimulating and highly enjoyable. As before, we have obtained feedback on the final draft of the book from an educator, a lay reader, a scientist, a doctor, and an expert in the field. Therefore we are pleased to have this opportunity to thank our colleagues for assisting us in taking this second edition of *Tourette syndrome: the facts* forward. Responsibility for any errors or inaccuracies remains, of course, entirely ours. We would like to reassure readers that the names of the individuals in Chapter 1 and Appendix 5 are entirely fictional.

London   Mary Robertson

March 2008   Andrea Cavanna

Preface to the first edition

Over the years hundreds of children and adults with Tourette syndrome, and their families, have attended our clinic at the National Hospital, Queen Square, in London. They have repeatedly told us of their need for a readable, slim text on Tourette syndrome, summarizing what is known about the condition for a general reader; hence this book. We have not included references in the text, so as to keep this publication as user-friendly as possible. Jargon has been reduced to a minimum. Where terminology is needed, we have defined it. For those who wish to delve further into the large literature on this subject, a bibliography is provided at the end. We hope that patients and their families, many of whom have helped us considerably in our research, will find this book of value.

London   M.M.R.

September 1997   S.B.C.

Acknowledgments

We are grateful to Tourettes Action of the UK and the Tourette Syndrome Associations/Foundations of Australia, Canada, Norway, and the USA for supporting our research, and also for assistance with this book and for supplying us with the names of several successful people who have TS about whom we were unaware. We are enormously grateful to Tim Howard and Pete Bennett for giving us permission to publish their photographs. We would like to thank Tim Howard's managers Daniel Segal and Mari Villalobos for facilitating communications between us and Tim Howard, and, as well as Dr Mort Doran, Kellie Haines, Dr Duncan McKinlay and Pelle Sandstrak, for supplying biographical details. Jeannette Page, Amber Carroll, Professor Roger Fenner, Dr Hugh Rickards, and Dr Helen Simmons read the penultimate draft of this book and gave us valuable suggestions for improving it which we much appreciate. The Bridgeman Art Library kindly supplied the photographs of Dr Samuel Johnson and Peter the Great of Russia. We would like to acknowledge Professor Simon Baron Cohen who co-authored the first edition with MMR. We would also like to thank the staff at Oxford University Press for their help. Finally, we are indebted to John Ludgate for his patience, support, and encouragement at every level.

Contents

1 Introducing three cases   1

2 What is Tourette syndrome?   13

3 How common is Tourette syndrome?   17

4 How is the diagnosis made?   21

5 What other disorders can be mistaken for Tourette syndrome?   31

6 Can people with Tourette syndrome also develop other conditions?   35

7 Will I have Tourette syndrome for ever?   43

8 Coping with the news of a diagnosis of Tourette syndrome   49

9 Is there more than one type of Tourette syndrome?   61

10 What causes Tourette syndrome?   67

11 Which therapies are most useful for Tourette syndrome?   75

12 Education, employment, and empowerment   83

13 Famous or successful people who have had Tourette syndrome   107

Appendix 1. An introductory card   127

Appendix 2. Bibliography   129

Appendix 3. Tourette syndrome international contacts and associations   143

Appendix 4. Feedback Form and Fact Sheet   153

Appendix 5. School letter   157

Index   161

1

Introducing three cases

⮕ Key points

◆ Tourette syndrome (TS) is a medical condition that usually begins in early childhood and persists throughout life. TS is characterized by the presence of multiple motor tics as well as vocal tics (noises), behavioural problems are common, and the condition is often socially stigmatizing.

◆ As TS can present very differently in each affected individual, covering a spectrum from very mild to more uncommon severe forms, this introductory chapter presents a few example cases.

Gilles de la Tourette syndrome (also known as Tourette's disorder, or Tourette syndrome, but mostly called TS for short) has been recognized as a medical condition for over 180 years. The main features include multiple *motor tics* (involuntary muscle movements), and one or more *vocal or phonic tics* (noises), which occur in bouts many times a day. The number, frequency, and complexity of the tics often change over time. They can be quite mild in some cases (slight facial tics and little noises, which some people might call 'habits' or 'mannerisms' (e.g. excessive blinking or squinting and repetitive sniffing), but in other cases can be very distressing and disabling, interfering with actions and speech (see Chapter 2).

The first clear description of the syndrome was made in France in 1825, when Itard documented the case of a noblewoman, the Marquise de Dampierre. Subsequently, in 1885, the French neurologist and neuropsychiatrist, Georges Gilles de la Tourette (Figure 1.1) working at the Salpêtrière Hospital in Paris, described nine cases of the syndrome, emphasizing a triad of multiple tics, coprolalia (inappropriate and involuntary swearing), and echolalia (involuntary

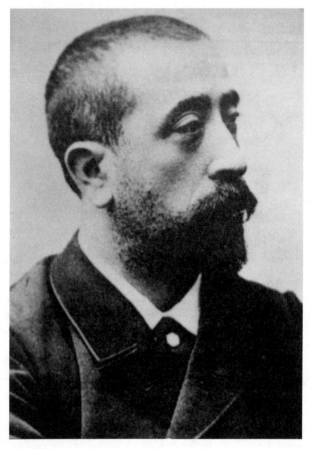

Figure 1.1 Gilles de la Tourette.

echoing back of the speech of others). British lexicographer Samuel Johnson, who compiled the first English dictionary, also had TS, as detailed in the writings of James Boswell. Present-day examples of successful people with TS include international level sportsmen, physicians, senior business people, and comedians (see also Chapter 13).

Originally TS was thought to be a rarity. For example, between 1825 and 1900 only 23 papers on the topic were published in the medical literature, the majority of which were case reports. An international registry published in 1973 reported only 485 cases worldwide. Since then, however, the literature has expanded enormously, and substantial numbers of patients are now documented. The prevalence (i.e. how common TS is) has now been documented to be 1per cent of youngsters (see Chapter 3).

TS can take many forms. For some people it may involve mild facial tics and a few vocalizations or noises that the individual may not even recognize as being 'different' from others. For other individuals, TS involves more dramatic and uncontrollable movements, and, for a minority, involuntary swearing as well. In other cases, symptoms may be accompanied by additional problems such as overactivity, poor attention, obsessional thoughts, and difficulties with impulse control. Because of this broad range of expression, we begin by describing three cases of people with TS, each of whom is typical but in a different way. Naturally, we have used fictitious names for them. In addition, these descriptions represent a combination of patients we have seen in our clinic, rather than specific people. Let us introduce you to them.

Johnny Thompson—a little volcano

Peggy and Peter Thompson were happily married. Peggy was an excellent dedicated teacher who had a flair not only for imparting information to children, but also for bringing out the best in them. She loved her pupils and they, in turn, loved her. Peter was a successful lawyer and a partner in a large prestigious practice specializing in patent law. Their only daughter, Laura, looked as though she was going to follow in her parents' footsteps. She was pretty, bright, popular at school, and succeeded not only in her studies, but also at her extracurricular activities and hobbies. She was, in fact, almost the 'perfect child'. Life in the Thompson household was almost idyllic. The atmosphere in the home was warm and happy.

Peggy and Peter had wanted another child for some time. They had tried and tried, but eventually, after medical consultations, Peggy was diagnosed as having 'secondary infertility'. Nevertheless, they were not put off, and kept on trying to have another child. After a couple of years they were delighted to discover that Peggy was pregnant. As Peggy was over 35 years old, an amniocentesis was recommended by the doctors, and to everyone's relief the results were completely normal. Similarly, Peggy had a scan—and again it was, thankfully, normal. On the scan it was clear that the baby was a boy, and even during the pregnancy the parents called him Johnny.

Johnny made himself known early on. Even during pregnancy he was on the go all the time, like a little volcano. He kicked and kicked and kicked. Peggy's initial dreams of Johnny representing England at rugby were soon replaced by her dreams for peace and quiet. At last the ninth month arrived, but after

2 weeks, Peggy went into premature labour. The delivery was assisted by forceps, apparently because Johnny was struggling despite his small size.

Peggy was sure Johnny was struggling because he was in too much of a rush—he just had to be born quickly! As soon as he arrived, Johnny began to cry—not gentle cries, but yells, as if to tell the world that he had arrived. Johnny continued to cry for what seemed like years. He cried during the day, but seemed to cry especially loudly at night, when others were trying to sleep. 'The crying drives me to hell and back', Peggy said to a close friend. Johnny did not sleep at night or take afternoon naps; he screamed for hours on end, hated being held, and would struggle to be put down.

However, despite these initial problems, Johnny seemed to grow and mature at a normal rate. He ate well, but failed to put on much weight. The doctor suggested that there was really nothing wrong, and theorized that the lack of weight gain was probably because Johnny was never still, and therefore was using up too much energy. He moved constantly in his cot, in his pram, and even in his high-chair. At night he seemed to move all the time, leaving his cot in a mess in the morning, with the sheets all over the place. He also started to bang his head in his sleep at night, which worried Peggy. Nevertheless, the family doctor continued to be reassuring; he said that many babies behaved like that and that Peggy need not worry. She tried not to.

As a toddler Johnny had temper tantrums up to three or four times a day. He would throw things and break them, and would try to hurt himself by banging his head on the floor or walls. The trigger for these rages was often something trivial, such as putting on the wrong shoe first.

By the time Johnny reached the age of the 'terrible twos', things were even worse. He made Peggy feel desperate. Peter was very supportive, but there was little that he could do. Johnny was irritable, impatient, and demanding, and could not take no for an answer. Life was exhausting. Laura, the older child, felt left out because so much attention was given to Johnny, but being such a placid and kind little girl, she accepted everything and seemed to continue to grow into a lovelier child.

The years went by. Johnny learned to talk; the only trouble was that he never seemed to stop talking, and he spoke in a very loud voice. He would butt into others' conversations, with no apparent regard for what they were saying.

When he started nursery school, it was a disaster, unlike Laura's experience there. Johnny drove the teachers to despair. Not only was he talkative, loud, intrusive, and even deafening at times, but he was also continually on the go. He was always out of his seat and seemed to have boundless energy. He had to hurry wherever he went.

Johnny had never crawled and now he did not walk; instead, he seemed to run and dash everywhere. He climbed on to things, jumped into things, and, in his haste, seemed to act without thinking. At junior school things got even worse. He was unable to concentrate, would sit gazing into space as if dreaming, and did not respond when spoken to. He often had to ask teachers to repeat what they had said. Johnny did not seem to understand instructions and started falling behind at school.

Things became so bad that Peggy took Johnny back to the family doctor. The doctor knew the family well and he appreciated that both Peggy and Peter were sensible, good parents. He also knew that they had been a happy uncomplicated family—until Johnny's arrival. The doctor found himself at a loss. Normally, when a child seemed so badly behaved, he would ask himself whether the problems might be the result of bad parenting or family troubles. In this family he knew that this was not the case. All he could do was reassure Peggy that it was part of 'growing up' and that, hopefully, Johnny would grow out of his awful behaviour.

But Johnny did not improve. Both at school and at home Johnny would make friends, but lose them as soon as they got to know him. He became isolated and lonely. Life was not a pleasure for anyone in the family any more. Johnny's behaviour began to get everyone down.

At about the age of 8 years, Johnny started to shake the hair out of his eyes excessively and blow his fringe. These activities persisted and became labelled as 'Johnny's habits'. His hair, especially his fringe, was rather long, and so Peggy took him to the barber to have it cut. The haircut made no difference—he continued to flick his head and blow, even though his fringe was now short. Then he began to screw up his eyes. The family doctor examined them and said that there were no problems with his sight.

Soon after, he began to stick out his tongue. Peggy and Peter reprimanded him, but that only seemed to make matters worse. He not only stuck out his tongue, but also began to grimace. He also started both to smell and to lick things, and occasionally he would spit—even in public. Life with Johnny became a continuous nightmare.

The family doctor was consulted again, and this time he referred Johnny and the family to a child psychologist. The psychologist listened carefully and, at the end of three assessment visits, was only able to say that she had never, in her professional career, come across a child like this. The psychologist raised the idea that there could be some family problems causing Johnny's behaviour. Peggy and Peter despaired. The next two years seemed to be full of constant noise and activity, with Johnny rushing about, apparently without thinking, not coping at school, having temper tantrums, and becoming lonelier.

Next Johnny began to repeat words and phrases he heard on TV, and would also repeat his own sentences or the last word of a sentence. He seemed distressed about his own behaviour even though, to others, it seemed deliberate. Peggy could not win; disciplining him did not seem to help, and ignoring the behaviour (in case it was attention-seeking) did not help either. She even thought that it could be caused by a food allergy, and so she did not allow him to have sugar, dairy products, red food colouring, or any food or drink with E additives. Still his behaviour remained unchanged.

At the age of 10 years, Johnny started coughing and making strange noises in his throat, as if it needed clearing constantly. Peggy took him to the family doctor again. This time he referred Johnny to a paediatrician. The paediatrician took one look at Johnny, took a brief history of the case, and pronounced that Johnny had TS with attention deficit–hyperactivity disorder, also known as ADHD. Peggy and Peter had never heard of such a condition, but when the paediatrician explained it to them, things began to fall into place. Only when the paediatrician enquired carefully and specifically into the family history did Peter remember that his father used to clear his throat constantly, and that his brother used to twitch his nose. The family had affectionately called this his 'rabbit twitch'. Both men were happily married, successful in their careers, and functioning normally. Their noises and twitches were so much part of them, and they were such likeable people, that the 'symptoms' had never really been considered abnormal.

Tourette syndrome—at last Peggy and Peter had a name for Johnny's problems and, with the diagnosis, hopefully some help. The paediatrician had only ever seen a couple of cases of TS but had seen many more children with ADHD. He decided to try Johnny on some medication—methylphenidate. It seemed to be magic for the hyperactivity (which decreased) and the poor concentration (which improved). However, the tics and noises became much worse and Johnny also began to lose weight. Nevertheless, because the ADHD and schoolwork improved, the paediatrician decided that this medication was better than nothing, and that Johnny should remain on it.

After another two years Johnny began to say 'fu, fu' and then cough afterwards. Then, one day, he said the full dreaded 'F word' in school assembly and was clearly upset at having done so. The family made an immediate appointment to see the same paediatrician, who recognized that the TS was worsening. He made enquiries in the medical world and decided to refer Johnny and the family to a specialist in TS. The specialist had seen hundreds of children and adults with the syndrome, which reassured Peggy and Peter at once.

The specialist took Johnny off methylphenidate, as it may have increased the tics and noises, and prescribed clonidine instead. Johnny's tics and noises slowly improved, the swearing became less frequent, and his concentration and hyperactivity remained under control. Life was never going to be easy with Johnny, but at least his behaviour was manageable. He began to catch up at school and even seemed to make some friends.

The specialist put the family in touch with Tourettes Action, from which Peggy and Peter derived great comfort. They realized that their story was not so unusual, and that Johnny was not a bad child; rather, he was a child in need of professional help, care, and understanding.

Now let's look at a different case of TS.

Tim—the teacher

Tim had had twitches and habits for as long as he could remember. At 5 years old, when he had just started school, he began to blink a lot and roll his eyes. He soon began to have head-nodding movements as well, which earned him the nickname of Noddy. At first his classmates teased him, and a few tried to bully him, but as he was temperamentally a fighter, he never let this get him down.

Tim came from an ordinary and happy home. His grandfather ran a small family business selling kitchen hardware. His parents were healthy and rarely visited doctors. Both his father and grandfather had had facial twitches and made repetitive throat-clearing noises when under stress. His father also said that when he had been at school, he had had problems with concentration. However, his intelligence was above average and he was a hard worker, which more than compensated for his occasional daydreaming. Tim had a brother and two sisters, all of whom had had no serious problems in their lives.

Tim liked school. He enjoyed learning and acquiring knowledge, and his ambition was to become a teacher. The nickname Noddy stayed with him through junior school where, after some initial problems with teasing and bullying, the name became a term of endearment. He was a likeable youngster and got on with most of the other children. When he was 13 he developed a strange tickling feeling in his throat and he felt compelled to clear his throat quite a lot.

He remembered thinking that he did not have a sore throat and he did not have a temperature or feel ill, and so it felt even stranger that he cleared his throat. Soon after that he began to cough for no good reason and this became a habit. Occasionally when he coughed more than usual, people would ask him if he was coming down with a cold or flu, but he always replied that he was fine.

Tim's tics and noises became a part of him. He was certainly aware of them. Before a tic he would feel a tension, a tightness, a tickling, or a 'prickle' in the area of the tic. He could stop the tics voluntarily, though this sometimes caused more inner tension. When this tension mounted up too much there seemed to be a rebound increase in tics after the periods of controlling his symptoms. Tim's tics waxed and waned—sometimes they were more or less obvious—but this seemed to be for no apparent reason. If he developed flu or a fever his tics seemed to disappear temporarily. The tic pattern would also change at times, with old tics disappearing and new ones developing.

Tim also had an urge to imitate or copy what other people said or did, especially people on television programmes. He imitated accents, words, and mannerisms. Eventually, these copied behaviours became part of his own behaviour, so that he was like a 'tic chameleon', absorbing and then reflecting the habits and noises of his surroundings. No one seemed to mind and it did not bother Tim. In fact, mimicking became one of his party pieces and a part of his developing character. At times he felt an urge to lick or smell things, but he realized the embarrassment that this might create, and so he was able to control the urge until he was alone. Then, when alone, he would smell or lick anything and everything in sight.

Tim was above average academically and did well at school. He was also good at sport, particularly soccer, and it was remarkable that his symptoms disappeared without any effort when he concentrated on sport. He went on to graduate from teacher training college and began to teach at the age of 22.

Occasionally, Tim liked to enjoy a pint of beer or glass of wine. He also had the odd joint of cannabis. Both the alcohol and the cannabis reduced the severity of his tics, but as his tics did not really bother him, he was never tempted to use these substances to excess. Tim had always had friends and girlfriends. His first serious girlfriend, Alison, was another junior teacher at the school. After dating seriously for 9 months they decided to get married.

Tim was in his third year of teaching when Cliffie, a new 9-year-old pupil, arrived in his class. Cliffie was a bright child, but difficult to manage as he was constantly on the go, jumping up and down in class, interrupting, and talking excessively. At times, Cliffie was also very inattentive. Tim noticed that, like himself, Cliffie had some facial 'habits' and made little noises such as repetitive sniffing. Tim thought that this was strange because, apart from himself, his father, and his grandfather, he had never really noticed facial mannerisms in other people. Cliffie proved to be a real handful in class.

Shortly after this, Tim and the school headmaster received letters from a doctor who provided a medical description of Cliffie. Cliffie's facial twitches, habits, and sniffing noises were described as being part of TS, and his hyperactivity was part of an associated condition, ADHD. Cliffie had been prescribed medication and the school was given strategies on how to deal with him. Tim asked his family doctor if he could be referred to the hospital himself, not because he needed or wanted treatment, but because he was curious about the apparent similarities (tics and noises) and also the differences between himself and Cliffie. The specialist met, interviewed, and examined Tim. He was indeed diagnosed as having TS, but it was so mild and Tim was so well adjusted that no medication was recommended.

Now let's look at our third and final case.

Annie's story

Annie Davis was a very special child. She was the only child born to parents in their forties. The pregnancy was normal apart from the fact that her mother, Kathy, was ill with excessive vomiting. The labour was normal in length, but Kathy was disappointed when forceps had to be used to assist in Annie's birth. As a baby Annie was very well behaved. She smiled early, much to the delight of Kathy and her husband Frank. Her early development was normal; she seemed to sit, crawl, walk, and talk at the same time as other children of her age.

Annie went to nursery school at 3 and managed the separation from her parents without fuss or distress. She was a naturally good mixer and particularly enjoyed playing with other children of her own age. She loved drawing, climbing on the jungle-gym, learning the alphabet, playing with plasticine, and doing sums. She laughed happily with her friends and when she went home in the afternoon she recounted her tales of fun to her mother.

Kathy was a part-time secretary. Her employer, a lawyer, valued her greatly, as she was extremely well organized, meticulous, and a perfectionist. She was able to accomplish in one morning what would have taken other people a whole day. Kathy ran her household with the same degree of precision. The home was decorated tastefully and well, all in pastel colours. Curtains and cushions were in the same fabric, ornaments were symmetrically organized, and everything 'had its place'. There were always fresh flowers in the dainty vase on the dining table and the wooden floor shone so much that it seemed clean enough to eat off! Frank was an architect. Although he was not as neat and tidy as Kathy, he appreciated her preference for arranging things neatly and symmetrically.

After a successful two years at nursery school, Annie began primary school. A bright child and still a good mixer, she adapted well once again. She was well above her peers academically and proved to be a good all-rounder. When she was 7 years old, Annie's class teacher noticed that she would squint and blink her eyes excessively. The teacher told Kathy about Annie's eye problem. Annie's health had been good so far and Kathy was shocked to hear of a potential problem. Annie seemed relatively unconcerned and reassured her mother that she felt no pain in her eyes. Nevertheless, Kathy was concerned, and so the family doctor was consulted and he suggested that soothing eye drops should be put into Annie's eyes three times a day. Kathy did as the doctor had instructed, but it made absolutely no difference. Annie did not seem particularly bothered but her parents were worried.

Kathy made an appointment for Annie to see an eye specialist. He put Annie through all the usual tests, such as looking into her eye with an ophthalmoscope, examining her eyes through a slit lamp, and getting her to read from a wall-chart. At the end of the examination, he said that Annie's eyes and sight were normal and there was no need to worry.

The school holidays began and soon Kathy noticed that Annie was blinking less often. When school started again it seemed as though the eye blinking had disappeared, but this behaviour was replaced by a stretching movement of Annie's neck, as though her collar was too tight. Annie said she felt a kind of itching and tension in her neck, although she had no pain. The family doctor suggested that Kathy rub a soothing cream into Annie's neck, but it made little difference. The neck stretching lasted for a couple of months, and then it too gradually disappeared. For a month or so, all was well.

Occasionally, Annie would make a facial grimace; she called it her 'funny face'. She would roll her eyes or purse her lips. As little movements or habits were now a part of Annie, Kathy tried to ignore them. The following summer Annie began to sniff and rub her nose at the same time. Annie did not look ill and certainly did not have any signs of a cold or flu. Kathy and Frank were puzzled and consulted the family doctor again. Perhaps Annie was allergic to something? The doctor prescribed some antihistamines in case Annie had an allergy. She took the pills for a month but they made her quite sleepy. However, the sniffing persisted and so Kathy stopped the tablets. Strangely,

Annie seemed relatively happy and unconcerned about her habits. Her school work progressed and she had friends.

Then something very different and far more worrying happened. When Annie went to the supermarket with her mother, she began to touch certain items on the shelves. Her touching rituals became more elaborate. Annie had to touch things exactly four times and when Kathy asked her why she did so, she simply said, 'I have to'. The touching spread into many other areas—at home, with friends, and even at school. Annie had always been popular at school, but when she began touching her classmates, their desks, their pens, and their schoolwork, they naturally began to complain. She also started to arrange things symmetrically. For example, if her place setting at the dinner table was not perfect, she would spend ages arranging the knife, fork, spoon, glass, and plate until they appeared totally symmetrical to her. She would become excessively concerned with the neatness of her bedroom and all her toys had to have their special places. She became very upset if any of these items were moved. When asked why she did it, she cried, 'I can't help it'.

Annie also began to have bathing and bedtime rituals. She would have to do things a certain number of times and in a certain way. If her routine was interrupted in any way at all, she would have to begin again at the beginning. A bath could quite easily take 30–45 minutes. Kathy and Frank were concerned not only that Annie now seemed unhappy, but that her touching and preoccupation with neatness and symmetry and her rituals had now become excessive.

Kathy went back to the family doctor who was baffled by the apparent change in Annie and referred her to a local child psychologist. The psychologist made an assessment and suggested some psychotherapy. Although Annie liked talking to the psychologist, it made no real difference to her various twitches, or indeed to her rituals. She was now 11 and the Davis family began to despair.

It was at this point that Kathy read an article in a magazine about a child with TS. There were many similarities between the child described and Annie. At the end of the article was the address of Tourettes Action. Kathy could not wait to tell Frank of her discovery. He agreed that the description of the child's behaviour in the article and that of Annie was very similar, so Kathy wrote to Tourettes Action. Their reply was just what Kathy and Frank needed—some literature on TS and the names and addresses of doctors who specialized in the condition. The family doctor was happy to refer Annie to a specialist as he himself had been baffled by her symptoms for some time.

The specialist neuropsychiatrist took a careful personal and family history, discovering that Kathy's father cleared his throat repeatedly and that he also had a number of habits. He examined Annie, reassuring everybody that, as expected, there were no serious abnormalities. He performed tests to rule out other more serious problems and, as expected, they were all normal. Annie was prescribed medication—a very small dose of sulpiride (for the tics) as well as fluoxetine (for the rituals and obsessions), the latter being in a relatively higher dosage. Annie was also referred to a psychologist specializing in cognitive-behaviour therapy, a special type of behavioural therapy, to help her reduce her ritualistic behaviours and 'habits'.

The neuropsychiatrist also reassured the Davis family that Annie's symptoms would diminish with the treatment and that she was otherwise a normal well-adjusted child. The only somewhat worrying aspect was that the TS was hereditary, and it appeared to have come from Kathy's side of the family. The prognosis proved to be quite correct. Annie's symptoms almost disappeared and she had virtually no side effects from the medication. Annie was once again a normal happy child.

Why are these three cases so different?

All three of the individuals described here have TS, but they differ in several ways. In Tim's case it is mild, not causing him distress and by and large not interfering with his life. Johnny, on the other hand, has TS more severely. His symptoms do interfere with his life and with those around him. Furthermore, Johnny has the accompanying condition of ADHD. Finally, Annie has moderate TS but with the accompanying condition of obsessive–compulsive behaviour. All three cases are typical but show different manifestations of the condition. Strictly speaking, the term 'typical' cannot be applied to TS. The expression of symptoms covers a spectrum from very mild, which is true of most people, to quite severe. It is not yet known why one person will show mild symptoms while another will demonstrate more severe symptoms and may have accompanying problems controlling his/her attention. However, it appears that TS probably should no longer be considered merely a motor disorder and, most importantly, that it is not a unitary condition (i.e. a single condition that is the same in all individuals), as was previously thought (see also Chapter 9).

2

What is Tourette syndrome?

➜ Key points

◆ TS begins in early life, usually between 5 and 7 years of age and consists of many tics.

◆ The syndrome includes motor tics or twitches and vocal tics or noises, which must have been present for a year although not necessarily together. These tics can be simple or complex.

◆ Vocal tics are often called phonic tics, as many of the noises made by patients with TS do not use the vocal cords.

◆ Common motor tics are blinking, head nodding, face grimacing, and nose twitching, and common phonic tics are sniffing, throat clearing, and coughing.

◆ The swearing tic (coprolalia) receives a lot of media attention but in fact only occurs in only 10–15 per cent of individuals with TS. In addition, there are differences between 'socially accepted swearing' and the swearing tic, which is involuntary, is often disguised by the individual, and causes embarrassment to the individual with TS.

What are tics?

TS is a medical condition of unknown cause, characterized by the presence of chronic muscular tics (movements) and at least one vocal/phonic tic (noise). A *tic* is an abrupt, sudden, and jerky repetitive movement or vocalization that involves discrete muscle groups. Tics often mimic a normal co-ordinated movement, vary in intensity, and are non-rhythmic. Tics are accompanied by intense *subjective experiences* (which the individual personally feels inside him/herself) variously referred to as 'premonitory urges' or 'sensory tics'.

They are experienced as irresistible but can be suppressed voluntarily for varying lengths of time, often at the expense of inner tension. In fact, the term 'involuntary', usually used to describe tics, can be confusing, as it is known that some people with TS do have good control over their symptoms. What is not recognized is that such control may merely postpone more severe outbursts of symptoms later on; characteristically there is a rebound of tics after prolonged tic suppression. Therefore people affected by TS often seek a secluded spot to release their symptoms after inhibiting them at school or work. Both motor and vocal tics may be classified as either simple or complex.

- Common *simple motor tics* include:

  - eye-blinking

  - shoulder-shrugging

  - facial grimacing.

- Common *complex motor tics* include:

  - jumping

  - touching

  - squatting

  - licking or smelling objects.

- Common *simple vocal/phonic tics* include:

  - throat clearing

  - grunting

  - sniffing

  - snorting.

Complex vocal tics mainly consist of uttering words or phrases out of context. Vocal tics should be more appropriately called phonic tics, as many of the noises made by patients with TS do not involve the vocal chords. Other complex tics, both motor and vocal/phonic, are discussed below.

Coprolalia

Coprolalia (the inappropriate and involuntary uttering of obscenities or swear words) occurs in about 10–15 per cent of individuals with TS, but may occur in as many as one-third of patients in specialist TS clinics. Coprolalia is quite different from swearing in a social context, as the words slip out against the will of the person, who will often try to cover their embarrassment (e.g. by coughing to disguise the swear word). It is rare in children or in mildly affected cases. There is some suggestion that it may be culturally determined, as in Japan it may be rare. If coprolalia occurs at all, it usually begins at around the age of 15, after the onset of motor and vocal/phonic tics.

Complex characteristic tics

Copropraxia (involuntary making of inappropriate obscene gestures, such as the 'V sign'), *echolalia* (imitation of other people's speech), *echopraxia* (imitation of other people's actions), and *palilalia* (repetition of the patient's own last word, phrase, or syllable) are characteristic symptoms of TS, and while they occur not infrequently in clinic populations, their frequency in mild TS individuals in the community is unknown.

Other symptoms, such as *mental coprolalia* (thinking obscene thoughts), *coprographia* (writing obscene words or phrases), and *mental palilalia* (silently saying to oneself the last part of a word heard) become known only when the clinician asks about them directly. These clinical features are not essential to make the diagnosis. However, they may be associated with TS and are explained more fully in Chapter 4.

Overall, the range of tics or tic-like symptoms that can be expressed in TS is very broad. The complexity of some of these symptoms is often perplexing to family members, friends, teachers, and employers, who may find it hard to believe that the actions or noises are not to be considered as voluntarily performed.

What factors affect tics?

The motor and vocal/phonic tics or noises may be aggravated and increased by anxiety, stress, boredom, fatigue, and excitement. In addition, some people have reported that premenstrual tension, some food substances (such as additives), and stimulants (such as caffeine, methylphenidate, pemoline, and amphetamines) may also make tics worse. In contrast, sleep, alcohol, cannabis, fever, relaxation, playing sport, dancing, driving, orgasm, or concentrating on an enjoyable task, such as reading, may lead to a temporary disappearance of the symptoms.

When does TS begin?

The average age of onset of symptoms is between 5 and 7 years old, with the most frequent initial symptoms being excessive eye-blinking, eye-rolling, or twitches of the mouth. Patients usually show more complicated movements later. These might include inappropriate licking, smelling, spitting, hitting, jumping, and squatting, abnormalities of gait involving posture and movement, and 'forced touching'. The onset of vocal/phonic tics usually occurs later than the motor tics, at an average age of 11, and usually takes the form of involuntary sounds such as throat clearing and sniffing.

3

How common is Tourette syndrome?

> ## ➜ Key points
>
> ◆ Until very recently TS was considered to be extremely rare.
>
> ◆ Reviews of more than a dozen large recent studies suggest that TS affects 1 per cent of young people aged between 5 and 18 years in normal mainstream schools, many of whom will not have been diagnosed.
>
> ◆ TS is much more common in people with learning difficulties, people with emotional and behavioural difficulties, people who require special education, and people with autistic spectrum disorders (ASDs), i.e. people with autism and Asperger's syndrome.
>
> ◆ Tics affect 7–28 per cent of young people.

What is the prevalence of TS?

The prevalence (how common TS is) and epidemiology (where TS occurs) of TS are more complex than was previously thought. This condition has had a long and complicated history as far as diagnostic criteria are concerned (Chapter 4), its changing and fluctuating clinical symptoms (Chapter 2), and the various contrasting and evolving theories regarding its causes (Chapter 10).

Until fairly recently, TS was considered to be a rare and somewhat bizarre curiosity. However, several types of study indicated that TS was *not* rare. First, the majority of patients who were examined by specialists in dedicated specialist TS clinics had family members with tics or TS, even if it was not severe, and they had not consulted a doctor. Therefore it was realized that TS was far from uncommon. Secondly, large families or *pedigrees* consisting of more than 50 members were studied and each had many affected relatives, the majority of whom had never seen a doctor for their tics. Thus a large but undetermined number of individuals with unidentified TS and tics existed in the community. Tim's father, described in Chapter 1, is an example of just such a mild case where a doctor has never been consulted.

More recently, one of us (MMR) reviewed the literature, and noted that two pilot (small exploratory) studies and 12 large definitive studies in mainstream and school-age youngsters in the community have documented remarkably consistent findings, suggesting that prevalence figures for TS range from 0.4 to 3.8 per cent for youngsters between the ages of 5 and 18 years. MMR calculated that 397 (0.95 per cent) of the 418 312 young people studied internationally were diagnosed as having TS. Therefore it was suggested that a figure of 1 per cent would be appropriate for the international prevalence of TS. Notably, in the majority of these studies, the individuals identified as having TS were *mildly affected* and probably *undiagnosed* previously. Nevertheless many of the individuals with TS who were identified in the studies had had some difficulties with education or behaviour. The senior authors in all of the studies had a special interest in TS, and the methods used included direct observations and examinations of the young people in the study. Therefore it is suggested that these figures and difficulties are representative of TS in the community in most parts of the world. TS appears to be much less common in African Americans and, if it occurs at all, is even less common in Sub-Saharan black Africans.

It is generally agreed that having a major psychiatric illness, such as schizophrenia, is *not* associated with TS. However, TS is over-represented in people with learning difficulties, 'mental retardation', behavioural difficulties, and autistic spectrum disorders (i.e. autism and Asperger's syndrome). For example, 6–11 per cent of youngsters with autistic spectrum disorders have been reported to have TS. Furthermore, individuals in special educational settings for people with learning difficulties (called mental retardation in some countries) have a higher incidence of TS.

Tic disorders, usually referring to motor tics, are much more common than TS, although prevalence figures differ depending on the population studied. They have been reported to occur in 7–28 per cent of children and adolescents, but are uncommon in the elderly (less than 1 per cent). Based on these figures, tic disorders are the most common movement disorder in childhood. They are also more frequent in those individuals with behavioural difficulties, those with learning difficulties, those requiring special education placement, and those seen as 'problem children' (sometimes it is difficult to say whether they are 'problem children' because of TS or vice versa, but nevertheless more of these problem children have TS than do other youngsters).

Why is TS diagnosed more frequently these days?

Prevalence and epidemiology depend, at least in part, on the *definition* of TS and the type of *methods* used to ascertain a diagnosis. For instance, many clinicians erroneously believe that coprolalia must be present for the diagnosis to be made, and therefore the diagnosis is frequently missed by inexperienced clinicians. Many patients with TS can also attract a wide variety of incorrect diagnoses before the correct one is made by an expert specialist.

The prevalence of *full-blown TS* as described by Dr Georges Gilles de la Tourette in 1885, including multiple tics, coprolalia, and echolalia, is unknown but it is certainly far less common than the disorder consisting of motor and vocal tics only (see Chapter 9).

Tics are multidimensional in nature:

◆ the intensity of symptoms can range from mild to severe

◆ the frequency of symptoms can range from rare to constant

◆ a variety of symptoms (single and/or multiple tic groups) can apply to each individual

◆ the complexity of tics can range from simple to highly complex

◆ other existing psychiatric disorders can be present in the individual (which in turn affect disability).

There is no diagnostic test for TS, and indeed no definitive diagnosis other than the clinical diagnosis (see Chapter 4). Factors that may hinder a diagnosis are:

◆ the varying methods of study employed to diagnose TS

◆ symptom intensity and frequency decrease with age

◆ affected individuals are often unaware of their tics

◆ comorbid (co-occurring) disorders may mask tics

◆ tics may reduce with the treatment of comorbid disorders.

These factors can complicate research further and represent possible explanations for differing prevalence figures.

Finally, nowadays there is an increased *awareness* of the condition among health professionals. Publications in the medical literature are frequently followed by radio, TV, and press exposure, and this media attention in turn increases public awareness. In some instances there may even be over-diagnosis by the medical profession. Tourettes Action in the UK, and the Tourette Syndrome Associations and Foundations throughout the world have also had a huge impact in increasing the awareness of TS among doctors and educators. However, worldwide, there are still a large number of individuals who remain undiagnosed.

Does TS occur universally?

TS affects individuals in all cultures and countries where it has been looked for. Although clinically it is a rather complex condition, its main characteristics seem to be independent of culture, highlighting the biological underpinnings of the disorder. In other words, the symptoms of TS occur with some degree of uniformity irrespective of the country of origin. The majority of studies agree that it is three to four times more common in males than in females. The disorder seems to be rarer in some ethnic groups. In the large review referred to earlier and in a study undertaken by Professor Mary Robertson, she suggested that TS may be rarer in Oriental people, is not common in the North American 'African American', and is virtually absent in Sub-Saharan black African people, i.e. other than South Africa. This may be due to either under-recognition or genetic factors (which we will discuss later). The disorder is also found in all social classes. Some research suggests that people with TS may be under-achievers. This under-achievement may be directly due to TS (e.g. the tics *per se*), or the stigma associated with it, or indeed the co-occurring disorders.

4

How is the diagnosis made?

Key points

- There is no blood test for TS.

- An expert will assess the individual by taking a history, examining the patient, and using rating scales completed by the doctor and by the patient to give detailed information on the tic history.

- Even in expert clinics the assessment is long, and may take 2–3 hours.

- Some doctors take blood tests or perform investigations such as an EEG to exclude other conditions.

A diagnosis is essential if different conditions are to be clearly distinguished from one another and is important in the understanding and treatment of such conditions. In the case of TS, early diagnosis offers the hope that management can begin before the syndrome pushes the individual too far off the normal course of development, resulting in problems with education, relationships, work, and career.

Because TS is not widely known, it may go unrecognized even in the twenty-first century. Indeed, many patients are diagnosed only when they reach adolescence or adulthood. It is hoped that with better education of both professionals and the lay public, earlier recognition and thus earlier diagnosis will take place. However, despite having heard of TS, some doctors are unwilling to make a firm diagnosis. For example, if a patient has 'only' motor and vocal tics or 'simple TS' (see Chapter 9), some doctors will not diagnose TS and merely call it a 'tic disorder'. Other doctors still labour under the misapprehension that coprolalia (involuntary inappropriate swearing) must be present for the diagnosis of TS to be made.

TS was once thought to be rare, but now it is being recognized and diagnosed increasingly often. In this chapter we describe an assessment format used at the Tourette Clinics of the National Hospital for Neurology and Neurosurgery and St Georges' Hospital in London, and at the Tourette Clinic of the Queen Elizabeth Psychiatric Hospital in Birmingham (UK). This format is basically similar to diagnostic methods used in other countries where there are also experts and specialists in TS.

How patients are referred to the clinic

Often parents bring their child to the clinic, having been referred by their family doctor. Initially, the parents themselves suspect that the child has symptoms of the condition. Their suspicions may have been aroused by seeing a television programme or reading an article about someone with TS. In many countries, family doctors or parents find specialist clinics through the national TS Association or Foundation (in the UK this has recently been renamed Tourettes Action), which keeps a list of doctors who are familiar with diagnosing and treating patients with the syndrome (see Appendix 3).

The diagnosis

TS is a *syndrome*, i.e. a disorder in which there is a clustering of a number of essential characteristic symptoms, which may include a number of other associated features and behaviours.

Motor and vocal tics

The essential features of TS are the presence of multiple motor tics (twitches) and one or more vocal or phonic tics (noises). The tics may appear simultaneously or at different times throughout the illness. Typically, the tics occur many times a day, in bouts, and must have been present for at least a year if a diagnosis is to be made. The doctor making the diagnosis will also check the age of symptom onset of TS, because this is usually before the age of 18.

The doctor will ask about the anatomical location of the tics (i.e. which part of the body they are in) and the number, frequency, complexity, and severity of the tics as they characteristically change over time.

Motor tics may involve the following areas of the body:

◆ head and face (e.g. excessive eye-blinking or squinting, eye-rolling, nose twitches, mouth opening, tongue protrusion, making faces, head nodding, or turning the head sideways)

- shoulders (shrugging)

- arms (jerking in or out)

- legs (kicking)

- abdominal contractions (pulling in the tummy).

Complex tics include smelling and licking things, spitting, touching of parts of the body, forced touching of objects, abnormalities of gait (such as funny walking and twirling), squatting, hopping, skipping, and bending down.

Simple vocal tics include sounds such as repetitive sniffing, snorting, throat-clearing, coughing, and gulping. *Complex vocal tics* include whistling, belching, and animal noises similar to a dog yelping or barking; duck and pig noises can also occur but are infrequent.

Other characteristic features

Concern need not be felt if the doctor asks about coprolalia (the inappropriate, involuntary, and often disguised uttering of obscenities and blasphemous words), as this must be explored. It occurs in about 10–15 per cent of individuals with TS. The full word need not be uttered, and so the doctor may ask if the patient says merely 'fu', or disguises the word and says 'fick', followed by a cough and covering of the mouth. Copropraxia (the inappropriate, involuntary, and often disguised making of obscene gestures such as the 'V sign' or 'third-finger sign') occurs in a few patients, and so again specific enquiries will be made about this.

Next, another set of symptoms will be specifically checked, including whether the patient demonstrates any of the following:

- echolalia—copying what other people say (e.g. repeating what they say or copying their accents)

- echopraxia—copying what other people do (e.g. copying their movements)

- palilalia—repeating oneself over and over, especially the last word or phrase said

- palipraxia—repetitive movements (e.g. doing up a button over and over again).

These symptoms occur in a substantial proportion of people with TS, but often have to be specifically enquired about. Not all symptoms occur in all patients.

Associated features and disorders

As will be described in more detail in Chapter 6, the most characteristic associated and integral symptoms are obsessions and compulsions. *Obsessions* are persistent ideas, thoughts, impulses, or images that are experienced as intrusive, inappropriate, senseless, and repetitive. *Compulsions* are repetitive behaviours (e.g. handwashing, ordering, checking) that are performed in order to prevent or reduce anxiety or distress.

Because obsessions and compulsions are disturbing for the patient, they are technically called 'egodystonic' (unwanted, intrusive, and uncomfortable for the individual). In obsessive–compulsive disorder (OCD), the common obsessions often have to do with dirt, germs, and contamination. The resultant compulsions have to do with cleaning and washing. Obsessional doubting, and therefore repetitive checking, are also common. However, in TS, the obsessions often involve thinking about violent scenes, sexual thoughts, and counting ('arithmomania'), and the compulsions have to do with symmetry, 'evening up', lining things up, and getting things 'just right'. To contrast it with OCD, many people refer to these behaviours in TS as obsessive–compulsive behaviours (OCB). These are often 'egosyntonic' (not uncomfortable but even sometimes pleasurable for the individual). If the doctor asks about these things, it is to check if the diagnosis should be of 'pure' TS, or TS with OCB, or even TS with OCD.

Attention deficit–hyperactivity disorder (ADHD) is characterized by poor concentration and attention, being easily distracted, impulsiveness, and hyperactivity. It is relatively common in people with TS, especially children, where ADHD may often cause disruption in the school classroom and difficulties with education for the child and his/her classmates. The doctor will again need to check if the appropriate diagnosis is 'pure' TS, or TS with ADHD.

Other distressing associated behaviours include non-obscene socially inappropriate behaviours (NOSI) and self-injurious behaviours (SIB), such as head-banging or body-punching, which can be dangerous. Examples of NOSI are commenting on others' weight, appearance, or personal characteristics in a way that is socially inappropriate (e.g. 'You are fat, aren't you'). SIB is seen in about a third of patients with TS and they hurt (slap, punch, hit) themselves not because they want to (they often do not) but because 'they have to'. SIB is significantly associated with obsessionality. This is in contrast with the 'self-cutting' of young women who cut themselves when they feel low, angry, or distressed, and often relieve these feelings by doing so. They may get relief on seeing the blood and there may also be a 'thrill'. In these cases, cutting occurs for complex reasons but *not* because they 'have to' (with an obsessional quality, as in patients with TS). Depression is also quite common in clinic patients with TS. Any of these associated behaviours will be noted and fully described in Chapter 6 because they will obviously have implications for management and treatment.

Nevertheless, it is important to realize that many people with TS are only mildly affected, live in the community, never seek medical attention, and may not be distressed by their symptoms.

The assessment

Although there are a number of different approaches to assessing individuals with TS, the basic principles are usually the same at different centres.

In the first place, a thorough *history* must be taken, enquiring specifically about the onset of tics and their progression, other characteristic symptoms, and the associated behaviours. In some clinics, specialized *interview schedules* are used to gather the information in a standardized way so as to make an accurate diagnosis, to be sure of enquiring about all the associated features, and to enable the clinician to make an accurate assessment of the severity of the symptoms. The history is usually taken from both the patient and another informant (e.g. parent, carer, spouse, partner, or teacher).

The clinician has to perform a *neurological examination* (examining the nerves and the muscle reflexes) because there are sometimes subtle abnormalities in TS, and also other neurological disorders need to be excluded. The clinician will then also perform a *mental state examination* to look for depression (which can occur in TS) and to exclude other psychiatric conditions, such as psychosis (e.g. schizophrenia or mania). This takes the form of some standard questions. It is important to exclude schizophrenia and mania as they can be treated, but it is not common to find them in association with TS.

There are many standardized physician and self-report rating scales or schedules that help in the more accurate description of symptoms. These are used by specialists and include:

- the National Hospital Interview Schedule
- the Yale Global Tic Severity Scale
- the Diagnostic Confidence Index
- the Motor tic, Obsessions and compulsions, Vocal tic Evaluation Survey (MOVES) Scale

- the Hopkins Motor and Vocal Tic Severity Scale

- the Tourette's Syndrome Videotaped Scale

- the PUTS Scale to examine the very specific premonitary urges of TS.

In order to implement the majority of these scales, familiarity with TS, as well as training by an expert, is important. Many of these scales are used in our clinics as they not only help to obtain accurate diagnosis (e.g. National Hospital Interview Schedule), but also give a likelihood of diagnosis (e.g. Diagnostic Confidence Index), indicate severity (e.g. Yale Global Tic Severity Scale, MOVES Scale), assess specific symptoms/sensations (e.g. PUTS Scale), and identify those that can be used in research protocols (e.g. Tourette's Syndrome Videotaped Scale). Standardized schedules are mandatory for research and are useful for accurately assessing the response to medication.

There are also several standardized self-report scales that help to give the patient's account of the associated psychopathology (psychiatric problems) or comorbid (co-occurring) disorders such as depression, anxiety, ADHD, OCB, and behaviour. These include:

- ADHD—Conners (parents and teachers)

- Obsessionality—Leyton (adults and young people)

- Depression—Beck (adults) and Birleson (young people)

- Anxiety—Spielberger (Spielberger State and Trait Anxiety Inventory, STAI)

- Behaviours—Child Behaviour Checklist (CBCL)

- Strengths and Difficulties Questionnaire (SDQ)

- Social Communication Disorder Checklist.

In terms of clinical diagnosis, special investigations are not useful if the assessor is experienced with the syndrome. Although the exclusion of Wilson's disease (a condition caused by abnormality of copper in the organism) with blood tests of copper and caeruloplasmin is considered mandatory, in the authors' experience no patient presenting with this distinctive picture of TS has actually had Wilson's disease and certainly more extensive investigation of copper handling is not necessary.

Usually no further tests are undertaken, but if there are atypical features, the clinician may refer the person for one or more of the following tests.

◆ An *electroencephalogram* (EEG), which is a painless investigation with no uncomfortable effects, involving fixing small discs to the scalp and recording the activity of the brain. The EEG can prove useful to rule out a diagnosis of a specific kind of epilepsy called myoclonic epilepsy. Scans are undertaken to exclude other less common causes of tics, including brain abnormalities.

◆ A *brain scan,* which may involve computed tomography (CT) or magnetic resonance imaging (MRI). In research, fMRI (functional magnetic resonance imaging) is also used. Positron emission tomography (PET) or single-photon emission computed tomography (SPECT) are usually only performed for research purposes.

◆ *Neuropsychological* testing (often involving IQ or intelligence testing) is not routinely performed, as the overall IQ is usually in the normal range in the child with TS. However, neuropsychological testing is mandatory in patients with learning difficulties and useful for research.

◆ An *electrocardiogram* (ECG), a test recording the activity of the heart, must be performed if certain drugs (e.g. pimozide, aripiprazole, atomoxetine) are to be prescribed, as abnormalities of the ECG can occur with these medications.

◆ In our clinics we often take 'baseline' *blood samples,* including tests for prolactin, which increases after certain medications (e.g. neuroleptics).

◆ We also measure the *baseline weight and height* of our patients as some medications can affect growth and/or appetite, and we also use growth charts to monitor height and weight.

More recently, specific blood investigations have been developed for selected patients. These include anti-basal ganglia antibodies titres, based on the hypothesis (or suggestion) that in certain cases development of TS may be linked to an abnormal immune reaction following repeated bacterial infections (see Chapter 10). However, the usefulness of these additional investigations for routine clinical practice is still under evaluation. Even though we have published research on these, we do *not* use them routinely, but only if we suspect that they may be increased in a particular patient.

Clinicians experienced in assessing and managing patients with TS are usually able to do a complete evaluation on an outpatient basis, when the assessment can last for 2–3 hours. Often a tea or lunch break will be included, as these tests can be tiring for the family and the patient. If the problems are complex or difficult, a period of inpatient assessment may occasionally be required.

It is ideal for clinics to be multidisciplinary and include a psychiatrist, neurologist, clinical psychologist, behaviour therapist, social worker, and educational psychologist. However, this may well be too expensive for most hospitals in the public sector. Sadly, many clinics are staffed by a minimum of professionals.

In our clinics in London and Birmingham, and in several collaborator centres worldwide, the patients and their families are routinely provided with a per-sonalized Feedback Form and Fact Sheet (see Appendix 4), explaining which symptoms they have, the medical names for the symptoms, the severity of their TS, and the associated behaviours. Current information about the causes and treatment of TS are also included.

Why is TS not diagnosed in infancy?

As we mentioned earlier, TS usually becomes evident at around the age of 7 years, with the onset of motor tics. However, some children first manifest with hyperactivity or OCB. The question then arises: Why is TS not picked up in infancy? At present it is rare to diagnose the condition before the age of about 5 years, and in many instances it is not diagnosed until considerably later.

There are a number of reasons for this delay. First, before the age of 5–7 years, the patterns of behaviour and history of motor and vocal tics may not be clear enough to allow a definitive diagnosis to be made. Secondly, children with TS may also have ADHD, and it may be that the ADHD is the main cause for concern and a focus on this may mean that the TS goes undetected. Thirdly, in most children with TS, there is a period of normal development and only later do the motor and vocal tics and associated behaviours develop. Fourthly, because of the tendency of tics to wax and wane and change over time, it may take some time for the doctor to obtain a complete picture of the symptoms. Finally, because children (and adults) often suppress their symptoms in the company of strangers, including doctors, the tics may not be seen or heard and therefore the diagnosis will not made.

As yet, there is no blood test that can be performed on the mother in preg-nancy, or on the child, which can confirm the diagnosis of TS. This contrasts with the procedure in disorders where a gene has been identified and blood tests can confirm a diagnosis (e.g. Huntington's disease). This also means that prenatal detection of TS is not yet possible.

A late diagnosis may also occur simply because parents (or adult patients) have little experience of the development and behaviour of 'normal' children, and hence they may be unaware that they or their child have a problem. Tim the teacher's case (see Chapter 1) was just such an example. 'All children have the odd tic, don't they?' is a common statement that we have heard. After all, no parents like to think that their child has a 'problem'. The GP or health visitor may also have difficulties identifying subtle symptoms of TS (e.g. mild tics), and instead feel that they are simply transient developmental problems. This is not very surprising, given that it is unlikely for one of these health professionals to see even a single case of diagnosed TS during their whole career. As a consequence, parents are often told, 'He'll grow out of it'. As mentioned earlier, it is hoped that, in time, primary health professionals will become better able to detect possible cases of TS and refer such cases to specialists at younger ages for suitable early intervention.

5

What other disorders can be mistaken for Tourette syndrome?

→ Key points

- The main disorders that can be mistaken for TS are transient tic disorder (tics lasting less than 3 months) and chronic multiple tic disorder (in which the individual has either motor tics or vocal tics, but not both for longer than a year).

- Disorders developing later in life after exposure to some medications give a picture similar to TS and are called 'tardive Tourettisms'.

- Because 'dystonic' movements can be seen in TS, dystonia may be mistaken for TS.

- Because a patient can have jerky movements with myoclonic epilepsy, the two disorders are sometimes confused.

- Other neurological disorders in which the patient can have movements may be thought to be TS.

Distinguishing TS from other conditions

The task for the clinician is often to decide whether the patient has TS or some other similar condition. Sometimes he/she has to decide whether both TS and another condition are present.

TS can be confused with a number of other conditions. For example, it may appear similar to any of the following

- *Transient tic disorder* (TTD), in which single or multiple motor and/or vocal tics occur for at least 4 weeks, but do not last longer than 12 consecutive months).

- *Chronic multiple motor or vocal tic disorder*, in which single or multiple motor or vocal tics, but not both, last for longer than a year.

- *Adult-onset tic disorder*, in which the symptoms are much the same as in TS, but the age of onset is in adulthood. There is often a precipitant, and the treatment appears to be more difficult. The prognosis (long-term outcome) is less clear.

- *Sydenham's chorea* (St Vitus' dance), a movement disorder that occurs more frequently in females, usually children; 75 per cent of cases are associated with rheumatic fever. Many years ago St Vitus' dance was diagnosed fairly often. Both Sydenham's chorea and TS involve involuntary movements and both are associated with obsessional behaviours.

- *Huntington's disease*, a movement disorder that usually begins between the ages of 30 and 50 years, but may occur in childhood, and that is associated with early behavioural problems and, later, dementia. There is usually a family history of Huntington's chorea. Both Sydenham's chorea and Huntington's chorea are characterized by choreiform movements. These are random, rapid, fleeting, irregular, dance-like, unpredictable jerks, which are non-repetitive and never integrated into a co-ordinated act. They tend to be aggravated by voluntary movements, stress, or anxiety, and disappear during sleep.

- *Tardive tourettism*, a syndrome similar to TS, which usually begins after high-dose long-term treatment with neuroleptics (e.g. haloperidol, or pimozide). This is difficult to treat.

- *Tardive dyskinesia*, a syndrome of involuntary movements, usually predominantly around the mouth, also following high-dose long-term treatment with neuroleptics (e.g. haloperidol or pimozide). This is difficult to treat.

- *Dystonia*, in which there is twisting of certain muscle groups, often the legs, which is usually crippling and progressive.

- *Spasmodic torticollis*, involving a 'wry neck', which usually begins between the ages of 30 and 50 years.

◆ *Wilson's disease*, which usually presents between the ages of 10 and 25 years, with characteristic signs in the eyes and liver, and with abnormal copper in the blood and urine.

◆ *Epilepsy*, when the patient may have seizures or fits during which they have jerking movements, usually associated with a loss of consciousness.

◆ *Myoclonic epilepsy*, which is a type of epilepsy in which there is muscle jerking, with no loss of consciousness.

Finally, some children with *autism* (a condition primarily involving abnormalities of language, social communication, and peer relationships, together with restricted repetitive patterns of behaviour) may have echolalia, abnormal postures, movements called stereotypies (such as hand-flapping), and obsessive–compulsive types of behaviour. Such individuals can be complicated by the fact that TS and autism actually co-occur in many individuals. Some individuals with learning disability (also called 'mental handicap' in some countries) can also have stereotyped behaviours. The set of conditions with which TS should not be confused is summarized in the box.

Conditions not to be confused with TS

◆ Transient tic disorder	◆ Dystonia
◆ Chronic multiple tic disorder	◆ Spasmodic torticollis
◆ Adult onset tic disorder	◆ Wilson's disease
◆ Sydenham's chorea	◆ Epilepsy
◆ Huntington's disease	◆ Myoclonic epilepsy
◆ Tardive tourettism	◆ Autism
◆ Tardive dyskinesia	◆ Learning disability

Other conditions and behavioural problems

We have already mentioned that a proportion of children and adults with TS have a history of childhood *obsessive–compulsive behaviours* (OCB) and *attention deficit–hyperactivity disorder* (ADHD). Quite often it is these behaviours, and not the motor and vocal/phonic tics *per se*, which are a matter of concern and warrant treatment, as they can impair the subject's health-related quality of life.

In addition, some children and many adults with TS who attend clinics have symptoms of *depression,* which also requires appropriate recognition and treatment in its own right. Children may also have *oppositional defiant disorder* or *conduct disorder* and, once again, it is these that may be the major cause for concern, rather than the motor and vocal tics.

Typical signs of *oppositional defiant disorder* include often losing their temper, very defiant behaviours such as excessive arguing with adults for no apparent reason or in response to only minor provocations, actively defying or refusing to comply with adult's requests or rules, deliberately annoying other people, blaming others for their own mistakes and misbehaviours, being excessively annoyed by other people, being over-angry and resentful, and being spiteful and vindictive to others. These behaviours must not be confused with excessive 'naughtiness', and must occur much more than in their peers and cause impairment in their lives. Some doctors refer to these behaviours as 'challenging' behaviours.

Typical signs of *conduct disorder* include bullying, threatening, or intimidating others, starting physical fights, using a harmful weapon, physical cruelty to people and animals, repetitive stealing and lying, destroying others' property, fire-setting, staying out at night, running away from home, and playing truant. Some children with conduct disorder grow up into adults with a *personality disorder* (e.g. antisocial behaviours such as robbery and severe aggression). It is these behaviours that may cause more problems than the motor or vocal tics. Firm (though kind) handling is required to try and encourage them to conform to the social norms of society and to make them aware of the consequences of not adhering to them. In our experience, the majority of individuals in the community with TS do not have these problems, although patients in the clinic may have them. This over-representation of people with problems in specialist clinics is called referral bias (see also Chapter 6).

It is becoming clear from our own research and experience in the clinic that TS occurs more in people with *autistic spectrum disorders (ASDs)*, which include Asperger's syndrome, autism, pervasive developmental disorder, and social communication disorder. It is often these disorders rather than the TS which cause more problems socially and from an education point of view, but if the TS can be treated it is important to diagnose it.

6

Can people with Tourette syndrome also develop other conditions?

→ Key points

The majority of patients with TS (about 90 per cent) have other problems such as:

- obsessive–compulsive behaviours (OCB) and obsessive–compulsive disorder (OCD)

- attention deficit–hyperactivity disorder (ADHD)

- self-injurious behaviour (SIB)

- non-obscene socially inappropriate behaviours (NOSI)

- subtle neuropsychological deficits

- depression

- oppositional defiant disorder (ODD) and conduct disorder (CD)

- personality disorders

- autistic spectrum disorders.

Obsessive–compulsive behaviours

It is currently recognized that most people suffering from TS also have additional behavioural problems. In 1907, Meige and Feindel, in *The confessions of a victim to tic*, described a patient with tics who also had OCB. It is now increasingly evident that there is a strong association between the two conditions, both in patients and in their family members. For example, one study found that patients with TS are disproportionately obsessional, and that this phenomenon is *not* due to having depression. Other studies have demonstrated differences between 'pure' or primary OCD and the apparently similar thoughts and behaviours, or OCB, seen in people with TS.

In classic OCD, the majority of *obsessions* (repetitive, senseless, intrusive thoughts) are concerned with worries about dirt, germs, or contamination, while the majority of *compulsions* (repetitive behaviours) are usually to do with excessive washing, especially of the hands. By far the majority of OCD 'sufferers' really do suffer from their obsessions and compulsions, which are *egodystonic* (unpleasant and uncomfortable).

In people with TS, in contrast, the obsessions are often to do with thoughts about symmetry and mental counting, and sometimes sex and violence, and the compulsions are more concerned with touching, checking, and things being 'just right'. They may also involve self-injury (see below and Johnny's case in Chapter 1). Thus obsessive–compulsive and ritualistic behaviours characteristically seen in patients with TS entail the feeling that something must be done over and over again, for example touching an object with one hand after touching it with the other hand to 'even things up' or repeatedly flicking the light switch on and off. Children sometimes beg their parents to repeat a sentence until it sounds 'just right'. Although many of these are egosyntonic (not internally uncomfortable and do not worry the individual), they sometimes are not, and the burden of these symptoms should not be underestimated in the latter. If a child with TS also has OCB, he/she may be very slow and pedantic in the ways in which he/she does things and thinks, and this may also be a disadvantage from an educational point of view. The pupil may have to go over and over homework or a task (to get it perfect), to the extent that he/she cannot even complete it and as a result fails to hand it in when required. The obsessions and compulsions in TS appear to be independent of the severity of the disorder. Most researchers now believe that some forms of OCB are *genetically related* to TS, as confirmed by several studies including one conducted by one of the authors (MMR) on a pedigree of 85 family members of a TS proband (patient presenting to the clinic).

Attention deficit–hyperactivity disorder

There also seems to be a link between *attention deficit–hyperactivity disorder* (ADHD) and TS. ADHD is certainly common in clinic patients with TS (recall the case of Johnny in Chapter 1). The characteristic features of ADHD are poor concentration, short attention span, being easily distracted, hyperactivity and impulsiveness. ADHD has been shown to occur in as many as 1–9 per cent of boys in the general population, depending on the country of study and the criteria used for the diagnosis. In patients with TS, as many as 50–60 per cent of individuals in some clinics have some form of ADHD. However, the precise relationship between the two conditions is complex and remains unclear. Several studies of children with TS have reported difficulties in attention, especially on more complex tasks including serial addition (keeping a running total in your head), block sequence span (keeping track of the order of doing things), the trail-making test (keeping track of a route), and letter cancellation tasks (keeping track of key items). Overall, these problems can result in disrupted schooling, contributing to their academic underachievement. There are now an increasing number of studies that indicate that children and young people who only have tics, i.e. 'pure TS' or 'simple' TS (see Chapter 9), are no different from their 'normal healthy' peers when various measures of IQ or cognitive function, behaviour and depression are undertaken. In most instances it is the ADHD and not the tics that results in behavioural and other psychological problems. ADHD is *not* genetically related to TS.

Self-injurious behaviours

Some types of *self-injurious behaviour* (SIB) have also been linked to TS and occur in as many as a third of TS clinic patients, but even individuals with mild TS in the community may exhibit such behaviours. The types of SIB seem to be similar to those found in people with learning disabilities (mental retardation), for example head-banging, body-punching, slapping, bodypoking, and banging themselves with hard objects. The majority of these behaviours may have an 'obsessive–compulsive' quality to them. The individual feels that they 'have to' hit, hurt, or poke themselves—even though they do not want to. Some of these behaviours have recently been suggested to have an 'impulsive' quality to them.

Non-obscene socially inappropriate behaviours

Some people with TS are known to make *socially inappropriate statements* or demonstrate what are known as *non-obscene socially inappropriate behaviours* (NOSI). For example, one of us (MMR) wears make-up such as cheek blusher, and most of her clothes have obvious shoulder pads. One patient with TS came up to her during a clinic and, tapping her shoulders (and obvious shoulder pads), said 'Mary Robertson is going to play American football'. Needless to say, there was a laugh, and when things had quietened down he pointed at her again, saying 'Mary Robertson's overdone the blusher!'. Once another patient said to MMR 'Big frown you've got' (MMR had actually not understood what the individual was saying!). These personal comments are clearly not the way that most people would talk to their doctor, or indeed anyone. We have another colleague, Dr Walkup, and when he stepped on to the podium to give a lecture, a person with TS shouted, 'Walkup step down!'. Another of our colleagues is very tall, with wide shoulders, and had longish hair and a substantial beard. A person with TS shouted at him at a TS meeting: 'Moose, you big f****** moose!'. People with TS may also make racist or sexist slurs—that is, saying the most inappropriate thing possible at the time. When this occurs the person with the syndrome is often embarrassed. In many instances, what is blurted out in no way reflects the person's true feelings or beliefs.

Subtle neuropsychological deficits

People with TS may also have subtle neuropsychological deficits that may be very difficult to diagnose but can indeed impair the individual with TS at school, in employment, and in the home environment. These can include *executive dysfunction*, which means that the person has difficulties with planning and organization, as well as inhibition of tasks, thoughts, and actions. Thus the individual may have problems with the initiation and completion of tasks, and often, as they cannot generalize, they cannot 'learn from their mistakes'. *Sensory integration dysfunction* may not be generally medically recognized, or indeed be a generally accepted diagnosis; however, it is a problem for many individuals with TS. In this case the person has an altered sensitivity (usually *hyper-*, but can be *hypo-*) to many sensory stimuli including smell (e.g. intolerance of strong smells, disliking new soaps), vision (disliking busy colourful patterns), touch (disliking tight collars, shirt labels, tight clothes), sound (upset by sudden or loud noises), and even movement (is often clumsy and uncoordinated). Others may have *social skills deficits* (miss social cues that are obvious to others), and some may also have *memory deficits* (in working memory, procedural memory, and strategic memory) so that they may appear to be 'all over the place'. Finally, many of our patients are now being suspected of having *dyspraxia* (weakness in the ability to co-ordinate and perform certain purposeful movements in the absence of motor or sensory impairments) and *dyslexia* ('word blindness', i.e. the letters of words appear back to front to the individual and so when they write, they write letters backwards: 'crepantrr' (carpenter), or 'Whom from did you get that letter' meaning 'From whom did you get that letter'). When these subtle deficits are added to the other problems outlined in this chapter, one can see how the person with TS may well have difficulties with education and employment (see Chapter 12).

Depression

Several studies have found that clinic patients with TS are more prone to depression than control groups. It has also been suggested that the depression is related to the duration of the condition. This makes good sense, as TS may be a chronic, often socially disabling and stigmatizing, disorder when the symptoms are moderate to severe. Nevertheless, symptoms of *depression* in children and adults with TS require appropriate recognition and treatment in their own right. Recent studies have shown that clinical correlates of the depression in people with TS appear to be the tic severity, the presence of echo- and coprophenomena, the presence of premonitory sensations, sleep disturbances, OCB and OCD, self-injurious behaviours, aggression, conduct disorder in childhood, and possibly ADHD. The depression in people with TS has been shown to result in a lower quality of life, may lead to hospitalization, and very occasionally may lead to suicide. The cause of the depression appears to be multifactorial. TS and depression are not genetically related. Patients with TS are often also more anxious when compared with the general population. We suspect that depression and anxiety are secondary to having TS. There is not much written about 'pure' anxiety and TS in the medical literature.

Other behavioural problems

Other behaviours that occur more often than one might expect in clinic patients with TS are antisocial behaviour, including aggression, conduct disorder, oppositional defiant disorder, and discipline problems. Indeed, these are often the reason for referral in the first place and can be difficult to manage. For example, young people diagnosed with *oppositional defiant disorder* show behaviours such as often losing their temper, defiant behaviours such as excessively arguing with adults for little apparent reason or in response to minor provocations, actively defying or refusing to comply with adults' requests or rules, deliberately annoying other people, blaming others for their own mistakes and misbehaviours, being excessively annoyed by other people, being over-angry and resentful and being very spiteful and vindictive to other people. As stated in Chapter 5, these behaviours must not be confused with excessive 'naughtiness', must occur to a greater extent than in their peers, and must cause distress or impairment in their lives. Some doctors refer to these behaviours as 'challenging' behaviours. Similarly, in young people diagnosed with *conduct disorder*, it is usually this condition that gives cause for concern, rather than the motor and vocal tics. Typical signs of conduct disorder include bullying, threatening or intimidating others, starting physical fights, using a harmful weapon, physical cruelty to people and animals, repetitive stealing and lying, destroying others' property, fire-setting, staying out at night, running away from home, and playing truant. Some children with conduct disorder grow up into adults with a *personality disorder* (e.g. antisocial behaviour such as robbery and aggression). Again, it is these behaviours that may cause more problems than the motor or vocal tics.

There are no specific medications for individuals with oppositional or conduct disorders, although recently some medications have been tried, marketed, and even licensed with some success, but almost all specialists agree that behavioural management is very important. In addition, firm (though kind) handling is required to try and encourage these young people to conform to the social norms of society, and to make them aware of the consequences of not adhering to them. Some doctors have access to specialists who undertake 'anger management', which helps these behaviours in some cases.

Personality disorders have been reported in up to 64 per cent of adults with TS, the most frequently encountered being borderline personality disorder. These are not usually diagnosed other than in a clinical research setting, as diagnosis takes a long time and has wide implications. There are no medications for these 'personality disorders' but they may make the individual with TS less compliant with medication and appointments.

Autistic spectrum disorders (so-called pervasive developmental disorders, including autism and Asperger's syndrome) have been found to occur more frequently in TS populations. Subtle neuropsychological deficits have also been reported in subjects with TS. Most people with TS have been assessed as having normal intelligence, although on IQ tests their non-verbal abilities may be as much as 15 points lower than their verbal abilities. Some sufferers also have specific difficulties in reading, writing, and arithmetic.

Some clinicians have suggested that a wide variety of psychiatric conditions, such as phobias, alcoholism, drug abuse, gambling, and eating disorders, are highly associated with TS. While some *clinic* patients with severe TS may demonstrate some of these, most people with the syndrome in the community are *not* psychiatrically disturbed in these ways.

Table 6.1 Proposed relationships between TS and behavioural problems.

Behavioural problems	Relationships with TS
ADHD	Common in TS but not genetically linked
OCB/OCD	Generally suggested as an integral part of and is genetically related to TS
Affective disorders	Multifactorial—possibly due to association with OCD and ADHD, rather than to TS *per se*
Schizophrenia	Rare—the association is by chance
Personality disorders	Relationship is unknown and more research is needed (possibly due to ADHD)

Finally, in our opinion there is no significant association between TS and schizophrenia, although several medications used to treat psychotic symptoms have proved effective for the treatment of tics via their action on the neurotransmitter dopamine (Chapter 11). The proposed relationships between TS and behavioural problems is presented in Table 6.1.

Clinic versus community samples

A Canadian, Dr Roger Freeman, and the International TIC Database Consortium (including one of the authors (MMR)) evaluated no less than 3500 patients with TS from 22 countries, and showed that only 12 per cent have no associated behavioural problems. More recently, a community study conducted by a Swedish group, revealed that only 8 per cent of patients with TS did not actually have any other diagnosis, and as many as 36 per cent were diagnosed with three or more other conditions. In our experience, the majority of individuals *in the community* with TS have these problems (but they often may go undetected), although the difficulties may be more obvious with patients *in the clinic*. This over-representation of people with several problems in specialist clinics is called referral bias. However, in general, whether in the hospital clinic, or at school, or in the community, only 8–12 per cent of people with TS have only tics, which may well prove to be a distinct subtype of TS (see Chapter 9).

In conclusion, a proportion of children and adults with TS have a history of associated behavioural problems. Quite often it is these behaviours, and not the motor and vocal tics *per se*, which are a matter of concern and warrant treatment. Recent studies have shown that health-related quality of life in patients with TS depends on a variety of problems and difficulties that go far beyond the motor and phonic tics (see Chapter 8).

7

Will I have Tourette syndrome for ever?

> ## ➡ Key points
>
> ◆ TS gets better with time in most people.
>
> ◆ Motor tics begin earlier than vocal/phonic tics.
>
> ◆ Tics usually begin at age 7 years, are worst between 10 and 12 years, and decrease after 18 years.
>
> ◆ Tics wax and wane, and also occur in bouts.
>
> ◆ Tics can increase during stress and 'life events'.
>
> ◆ The worst obsessive–compulsive disorder (OCD) symptoms occur later than the worst-ever tic period.
>
> ◆ Quality of life may be decreased in adults with TS.
>
> ◆ Caregiver burden (looking after a child with TS) may be increased in TS.
>
> ◆ Older adults will always 'have' TS—even if the tics no longer bother them.

When does TS normally start?

As we have seen, the generally accepted international diagnostic criteria for TS include multiple motor tics and one or more phonic (vocal) tics or noises, lasting longer than a year. In addition, the age at onset of TS ranges from 2 to 21 years. In the natural history of TS, the motor tics often begin between the ages of 3 and 8 years, some years before the onset of the vocal or phonic tics or noises. A mean or average of 7 years is most commonly reported. The onset of the phonic tics is often about 11 years. It is important to remember that the tics characteristically wax and wane in terms of severity, intensity, and frequency. It has been reported that the age of 'most severity' is at around 10–12 years. Coprolalia (the swearing tic) which, as we have said, is uncommon, occurring in only 10–15 per cent of all patients with TS, often begins at around 15 years, but we have indeed occasionally seen it in young children.

What happens to the symptoms of TS with increasing age?

The first patient with TS was the Marquise de Dampierre who saw Dr Itard in 1825 and then saw Dr Georges Gilles de la Tourette in 1885—she must have been over 80 years old, and her tics were as severe as ever. Therefore it was initially thought that TS was lifelong, but several relatively recent studies have indicated that the symptoms reduce with age. Other research doctors have shown that at baseline at the start of the course of their disorder (and study) some 88 per cent of patients met threshold criteria for at least mild symptoms, but only 30 per cent met criteria for impairment or having difficulties with functioning because of their TS. At a 2-year follow-up, 82 per cent of the subjects met criteria for tic persistence, which was interesting in that there was no significant difference from baseline, but only 14 per cent met criteria for TS-associated impairment, which was significant. This meant that although the individuals still had their tics, they were no longer troubled by them and they did not cause any living problems. The most recent follow-up study used a rigorous design in which the researchers reviewed the first assessments of their patients with TS (aged 8–14 years): they had originally (between 1978 and 1991) been videotaped for 5 minutes according to a strict protocol. Follow-up videos of the patients were then made. A 'blinded' video-rater (he/she did not know whether the videos were the original or follow-up) assessed the video tapes and compared them for tics as well as a tic disability score. Results showed that 90 per cent of the adults still had tics. Many adults who had suggested that they were tic free were incorrect, as no less than 50 per cent had objective evidence of tics. The tic disability score reduced significantly with age, and only 13 per cent of adults received medication for tics compared with 81 per cent of children. The authors (Drs Pappert, Goetz, and others) concluded that although tics improve with time, they are persistent in most adults.

Another study examined children aged 14 or less and then again after 7.6 years and reported that 85 per cent had a reduction in tics during adolescence: only increased tic severity in childhood was associated with increased tic severity at follow-up. The average age of worst tic severity was 10.6 years. Overall, worst-ever OCD symptoms occurred approximately two years later than worst tic severity; increased childhood IQ was associated with increased OCD severity at follow-up. No more than about 20 per cent of children continue to have impairment and poor functioning by the age of 20 years. However, it must be remembered that TS that does persist into adulthood may be associated with severe symptoms such as self-injurious behaviour and severe coprolalia or copropraxia.

Tics occur in bouts

Tics often seem to occur in bouts over timescales of days to years. These bouts are characterized by brief periods of what have been called 'stable inter-tic intervals', which may last from just minutes to several hours or to even longer periods of time. It has also been suggested by Dr Leckman, an expert in the USA, that the waxing and waning of tic severity over the course of several months and the 'peaking' of 'worst-ever' tic severity early in the second decade (aged 10–12 years) may reflect the same *multiplicative* processes that govern the timing of the appearance and disappearance of tics.

The severity of the tics is affected by environmental factors

While we consider these facts, we must remember that the tics of TS can be sensitive to all sorts of factors such as stress, anxiety, excitement, and fatigue, which are known as environmental factors. Thus, even though a person's tics may have reduced substantially by the age of 18 years, they may for example go to university and take examinations or indeed move house or get married, or have any of a number of what are called 'life events' and their tics may then get worse. In the same way we often note that playing a musical instrument, playing sport, running, dancing, and driving a car reduces tics. Therefore some people perform more of these activities specifically to reduce their tics, particularly at times when they know that they may get anxious.

The effect of TS on the patient and family

As will be seen in Chapter 8, there have been studies showing that the quality of life (QoL) of adults with TS was significantly worse than that in the general population. The factors that influenced the QoL domains in patients with TS were unemployment, severe tics, obsessive–compulsive behaviours (OCB), anxiety, and depression. In a similar, but separate study, the 'caregiver burden' was examined for parents of youngsters with TS, and it was shown that parents of children with TS experienced psychiatric problems and greater caregiver burden compared with parents of youngsters with asthma. In other words TS can take its toll on the patient and his/her parents.

As doctors we take all this into account. Thus tics in TS probably decrease with age in the majority of individuals, but the symptoms of OCD/OCB may in fact increase. The adult with TS if unemployed, or with severe tics, OCB, anxiety and/or depression, may have a reduced QoL. We have also described how TS is genetic—and an adult with TS may also have a child with TS with all the problems that parenthood may bring, such as an increased caregiver burden and risk of psychiatric problems. Thus we are saying that even though the tics often reduce with age, other factors may affect the individual with TS as he/she grows older.

The prognosis (long–term outcome) of TS

As described above, although the prognosis of TS is better than originally thought with regard to tic symptomatology, the psychopathology, such as OCD, may persist severely until later in the individual's life. The course of TS is not what it was originally thought to be, and appears to be remitting. Therefore if an individual is examined at different times in his/her life, the clinical picture of TS may well be different. What is also interesting is that all of us TS doctors have had patients who have spontaneous remissions, i.e. they have got better, and this improvement appears to have had little to do with the TS symptoms, the medication, or the patient's current lifestyle. One thing for sure is that people do not die of TS—they die of other disorders, such as heart disease, cancer, chest problems, strokes, and other serious diseases, which have got nothing to do with TS.

However, many people with TS do not know that they have it, as their symptoms are so mild—even as adults. In addition, even if one has quite marked TS as an adult, it does not have to be a barrier to happiness. Just read chapter 13 to see what we mean.

In conclusion, even though the TS *symptoms* decrease with age, the individual will probably *still have TS as they grow older* (as their biochemistry, their genotype, and their gene(s) are the same), and so we suggest not only that the overall prevalence rate of TS is >1 per cent (i.e. adults and young people), but older people will always 'have' TS, even if it does not bother them, which in most cases it probably will not.

❌ Myths about TS

- TS gets worse with age.

- All people with TS have coprolalia.

- People die of TS.

8

Coping with the news of a diagnosis of Tourette syndrome

➔ Key points

◆ Many people feel relieved by the diagnosis as it empowers them and gives them an identity and a voice.

◆ In addition, many parents feel that they have been blamed for their child's behaviour and so the diagnosis of an identifiable disorder, TS, relieves them of any fault.

◆ While some feel the diagnosis is a blow, as TS is often given unsympathetic coverage in the media, most individuals realize that there is help with the symptoms and with education.

Background

To discover that your child has a condition that may result in potential lifelong disability is, naturally, a tremendous blow. When parents finally realize that their child has TS, and that it is not 'just a difficult phase he's going through', they may feel as if they have 'lost' the 'wonderful and normal' child they thought they had and they may be overwhelmed by a wide range of emotions—sometimes despair and depression, as well as anxiety about their child's future.

At times a cloak of guilt can envelop them, making them feel in some way responsible for their child's condition: 'Was it in my genes?', 'Was it bad parenting?' On occasion, they may feel a pervasive sense of shame or embarrassment because of the perceived opinions of others: 'They've failed as parents. Listen to their child swearing! And he's so young.' While noticing that the child is swearing is an accurate observation, of course it does not mean that they have failed as parents, because the child's condition is no-one's fault. All these emotions are understandable reactions to the stresses and disappointments induced by the child's developmental problems, tics, noises, and at times erratic behaviour. Similarly, when adults receive a diagnosis there may also be a variety of conflicting emotions. There may be anger, with the obvious question: 'Why me? Why us?'

Emotional reactions following the discovery of disabling conditions in general

A fair amount is known about how parents respond to the discovery that their child has a disability. The following account is a description of the type of feelings that immediately follow when parents are told that their child has a medical condition such as autism, Down syndrome, epilepsy, or cystic fibrosis. We begin with this description because it best illustrates the range of feelings and thoughts that can occur in these circumstances. However, many of these conditions are life-threatening, which is not the case with TS (see Chapter 7).

As TS is very different from all these other conditions, the description of the reaction to the above diagnoses is followed by an outline of the reaction to the discovery of TS, which is often different.

Not surprisingly, the immediate reaction to being told that one's child has autism, Down syndrome, epilepsy, or cystic fibrosis is sometimes similar to that seen following bereavement—an initial phase of *shock* and *disbelief* (parents sometimes talk of feeling numb or cut off from the world). To some extent, the numbness helps prevent parents from being overwhelmed by their distress, and seems to act as a means of buffering them from the full significance of the discovery.

Understandably, parents find it difficult to assimilate new information during this period, and they may need to go through things several times at a later stage to grasp them fully. As a consequence, doctors should try to keep information short and simple when initially discussing the diagnosis, and then go through the details when parents have had a chance to recover from hearing the news. As described already, we routinely hand out a very simple fact sheet and suggestions for further reading so that parents or patients can take it home, absorb the facts, and ask relevant questions at their next appointment.

The early shock may be followed by a period of *denial*. Denial may be the mind's way of keeping anxiety and stress at bay. In its most pronounced form, it may result in people acting as if nothing has occurred, but usually it leads to parents minimizing the seriousness of the conditions and fantasizing that their child will somehow be magically 'cured' or grow out of it.

The next phase of the reaction is often full of feelings of *anger* and *guilt*. Anger at the injustice of the tragedy ('How could this happen to me?' 'What have I done to deserve this?' 'Why my child?'), and guilt ('What did we do as parents to cause this?') turning to sadness and despair ('How can we ever cope?'). Finally, most parents adapt and become able to form a *realistic picture* of the problems, as well as of their child's strengths, and begin to focus on practical ways of coping.

The above account is based on the reactions most often observed when the parents' discovery of the disability is sudden, as might typically occur, for example, following the birth of a child with a severe mental or physical disability.

Emotional reactions following the diagnosis of TS

The types of feelings parents experience following the diagnosis of TS may be rather different. Very *few* parents in our clinics have the emotions outlined above. This is quite surprising, since TS, when severe or worrying enough to get as far as a specialist clinic, is in fact a diagnosis which means that the child is not 100 per cent 'normal'.

In the first place, the child with TS is actually born a 'normal child'—he/she looks normal and indeed behaves 'normally' for a long time, years in fact. As we have said, the tics only begin between the ages of 5 and 7 years. Therefore the parent gets to know the child without any disability or disorder.

Although there may have been pre-existing concerns about a child's development, TS may not be diagnosed until the child is at least 8 or 9 years old, and often much later (even up to their twenties). As a consequence, many parents already suspect that something may be wrong, so that the news that their child has TS does not come as such a shock, particularly when the siblings appear 'normal'. Nevertheless, even when parents have suspected it, the final confirmation of the diagnosis can still come as a hard blow. 'I'm so shocked', said a father recently. He and his wife had been seeing specialists for about three years as their son's diagnosis was very complex, but the final and definite confirmation of TS (with attention deficit–hyperactivity disorder and conduct disorder, in that case) was extremely upsetting for them.

However, another reaction, which is more common, is one of *relief*. 'At least the condition has a name and it proves that my child is not "bad" or "mad"', said a mother recently. Her child had been going from specialist to specialist and undergoing many investigations. All had proven negative and his conduct was therefore dubbed 'a behavioural problem'. The relief for this family was that he was not, in fact, 'a bad boy'—he just could not help his symptoms.

Many parents feel relief for another reason. Children with TS look normal, and have no particular facial characteristics or features. Therefore most people assume that they are normal and are just badly behaved, often blaming the 'frazzled' parents for rearing the child badly. The parents often say 'At last we can tell people that our son has a recognizable condition', and feel that they are less likely to be blamed. TS is not due to bad parenting and the parents are grateful to be told. This, in turn, is empowering for the parents.

However, another family reacted very differently. When young John was diagnosed as having TS, and we explained that it was due to dopamine malfunctioning or 'going wrong' in a certain area of the brain, the parents were horrified. 'Please don't tell us he's mad', they begged. We had a lot of work explaining how TS was *not* a sign of 'madness'. Although dopamine is also involved in schizophrenia (and indeed medications that are given for schizophrenia and TS, although in different doses, both block dopamine), TS and schizophrenia are *not* related (see Chapter 6).

Other factors may also affect the way in which parents react. For example, the severity of the motor and vocal tics or noises of TS, and the degree of accompanying behavioural disturbances may influence how they respond to the news.

In addition, the psychological resilience of each parent, and the amount of support available from their family, friends, and health professionals will also be important, helping some parents to pass through certain stages in their emotional reaction to the diagnosis more quickly than others.

Different people may pass through the stages described above at different rates or in a different order. Family members can help each other by showing their feelings. Couples may find it helpful to set aside regular times when they can discuss their worries, frustrations, and sadness together. Brothers and sisters may be jealous of the extra attention and time being devoted to the sibling with TS, not understanding that he/she is basically 'unwell' at some level. For instance, if a classmate at school swears, he/she gets into trouble. The child's sibling might well wonder 'Why does my brother or sister not get into trouble for swearing, but just gets attention?'. This situation is difficult to explain to a young brother or sister, but parents should try patiently to do so. Some siblings become sensitive brave advocates for their brothers and sisters with TS, both at school and in the world outside the family.

What is also important is that we may diagnose the child or young person, but then also elicit symptoms of TS, tics, or obsessive–compulsive behaviours in other family members, often the parents. This involves telling them that they also carry the genetic vulnerability—and so it becomes a 'family diagnosis' instead of just only the patient—proband (person presenting to the doctor) diagnosis. We always ensure that blame in no way plays a part and, by and large, families leave our clinics relieved and comforted.

Extreme reactions

Sometimes individuals get 'stuck' in certain stages of coping with news such as a diagnosis, or miss some out altogether, and this may lead to difficulties. Thus parents who cannot accept their child's medical condition may embark on a relentless search for a 'cure' by constantly seeking opinions from many specialists, but never feeling satisfied with the outcome. Continued searching for what might help the child is, of course, both important and valuable. However, extreme reactions are often based more on the parents' need to stave off the sad reality of their own plight, rather than on the child's needs. We have seen a few patients in our own clinics, or indeed in our collaborators' clinics, whose parents indeed undertake 'medical shopping' and peregrinate from doctor to doctor, always searching for a 'cure'. Thankfully these are the exceptions. A few patients' parents 'want to take their children to America', thinking that doctors there know much more about TS. The parents are so desperate for 'better news' that they forget that America is a long way away, and therefore regular follow-up would be very difficult as well as expensive because of the need to pay for treatment: the majority of UK TS specialists work for the NHS.

Other parents may be caught up in an unresolved phase of anger, becoming embroiled in protracted legal battles with professionals whom they hold somehow responsible for their child's medical condition. Again, valid legal redress is important; but extreme reactions are often based on the need to 'blame' someone. Some may respond by asking the specialist if he/she thinks that the previous doctors who failed to diagnose their child as having TS were guilty of medical negligence. Our opinion is that usually they are not. For a doctor not to diagnose a condition that is not well recognized or understood is indeed *not* negligence. Sadly, medical students at the majority of medical schools in the UK still do not have curriculum-based teaching about TS.

Distinguishing between normal and extreme emotional reactions to the diagnosis is not always straightforward. The distress and feelings of sadness that some parents experience may occasionally precipitate a severe depression in a predisposed individual. By depression we do not mean ordinary feelings of sadness, but rather a depressive illness—a profound misery, with frequent crying, and an inability to derive pleasure from activities that would normally be enjoyable. Often, such depression also involves feelings of pessimism, worthlessness, and excessive guilt, as well as disturbed sleep and appetite, and may be accompanied by feelings of weariness and low energy. Parents may also experience difficulty in concentrating or paying attention and feel a sense of numbness, leading to a vicious circle of guilt as they are aware of their child's need for attention and affection, yet they sense that the child knows that they are unable to supply it. If this occurs, parents may benefit from professional help, in the form of either counselling or antidepressant medication, or both. If this is a problem for you or your partner, you should ask your family doctor for help.

As we said earlier, most parents make a remarkable adaptation to the needs and problems of their child with TS. Actually, the process of trying to understand their child's problem often brings with it a special intimacy, which comes from the feeling that this is a special child who needs far more than most children and with whom one can develop a unique relationship.

Effects on the marriage or relationship

Given the added pressures of raising a child with a condition such as TS, it is small wonder that people often say that having a child with a disability makes or breaks a marriage or relationship. Therefore it may be reassuring to learn that parents of children with TS are probably no more likely to separate and divorce than parents of children without disabilities. Nevertheless, difficulties in the relationship may arise, and when this happens it is important to tackle them. Often no more is required of the parents than to set aside time for themselves as partners (rather than just as parents) when they can talk openly, and share and discuss difficulties and disappointments. To find time to do this may not be easy, but the time is well worth the investment. If it is a problem to arrange for friends or relatives to help with childcare, the parents should discuss this with one of the professionals.

Another problem in the relationship may occur if one side of the family is blamed for carrying the 'Tourette gene'. This accusation can be very harmful to a relationship. If there were any problems in the parental relationship beforehand, they may be exacerbated as one parent, in despair, blames the other for 'giving' the child the 'bad gene'. This is, of course, not helpful. None of us can choose which genes we pass on to our children, and inheritance involves many unpredictable factors. Nevertheless, when we are at the end of our tether we can say things that we later regret. It is often said that in despair, you may hurt those who mean the most to you.

Effects on other children in the family

If there are other children in the family, parents will have to tell them about their brother's or sister's TS. Precisely what is said will depend on the age of the particular child and his/her ability to grasp the information. The news may also be a source of distress to them and will need to be shared in a sensitive manner. It is important to pace what you say, so that your child is able to take the news on board and come to terms with it. It is not enough to have a one-off 'heart to heart' talk and then leave it at that. There will be a host of questions that young people will have about the problems of having TS. Parents should discuss these issues openly, to prevent children 'bottling up' their feelings and questions. Ideally, parents should strive to set aside time for siblings so they know they can ask any questions that are on their minds.

At present not much is known regarding the longer-term effects on development for siblings of children with conditions such as TS, although it does seem that the effects need not be negative, and indeed may be positive. Thus some of the research in this area has indicated that siblings of children with disabilities may develop a deeper understanding of people and of medical conditions in general; they may show more compassion and have a better appreciation of their own good health than do their peers.

On the other hand, some siblings seem to have problems in emotional adjustment and well-being. This is all the more so, as they may mistakenly fear 'catching' the syndrome from their brother or sister, and of course they are more at risk of inheriting the TS spectrum than a member of the general population. Siblings also have their own needs and, as far as possible, need time given to them to foster their own development. Parents need to be particularly alert to any hesitation that their other children have in inviting friends home. With younger children, it may be sensible for parents to talk to schoolfriends' parents to pave the way for having the friend to visit.

From our experience in the clinic, we understand that both children with TS and their brothers or sisters are particularly vulnerable to bullying and teasing. TS is an easy target for bullying, by the very nature of the condition. We know young patients who are cruelly laughed at and called 'Noddy' at school (just like Tim in Chapter 1), which, needless to say, saddens them greatly.

There is also an added pressure on siblings to protect their brother or sister from bullying or teasing.

Effects of TS on the quality of life of the individual

What has been not well researched is the effect of TS on the patient or the family. Only two studies, from our group in fact, have formally investigated quality of life (QoL) in adults with TS using standard measures. In the first, it was demonstrated that patients with TS showed significantly worse QoL than a general population sample. However, patients with TS had a measurably better QoL than patients with intractable epilepsy. The factors associated with a higher risk of poor QoL in patients with TS were unemployment, severe tics, obsessive–compulsive behaviours, anxiety, and depression. The second study showed that several domains were impaired in people with TS, including psychological aspects and physical, cognitive, obsessional, and social domains (also see Chapter 1).

Effects of TS on the parents of a young person with TS

Another study from our group evaluated the 'caregiver burden' and TS, examining parents for their psychiatric well-being. The study investigated the mental health and caregiver burden in parents of children with TS compared with parents in a paediatric asthma hospital outpatient clinic. Of the parents of children with TS, 76.9 per cent achieved 'caseness' on GHQ-28 (a general health screening instrument) compared with 34.6 per cent of the parents of children with asthma, and this effect remained significant after controlling for demographic variables. Parents of children with TS also experienced greater caregiver burden, and this burden was significantly correlated with GHQ 'caseness'. It was concluded that parents of children with TS are at risk of psychiatric problems (also see Chapter 7).

Telling a child with TS about his/her condition

Many children with TS may ask why they are different from other children, and parents may have to explain to them that they have a problem, what this means, and how it affects their lives. This is no easy task. Broadly speaking, the approach that we have advocated for siblings is also appropriate here. For a start, parents need to be aware of the issues, provide a suitable forum for discussion, share information at a pace appropriate for their child, and pitch the content of what they say at a level that can be understood.

Understandably, children who recognize their disabilities may become troubled by their condition as its impact on their lives becomes more evident. This may occur when the child is young, but usually happens during adolescence and early adult life when problems may arise in establishing and keeping friendships. Marked unhappiness (and even depressive illness) may occasionally develop as a consequence. If this does emerge, parents should seek professional advice for their son or daughter. A few children with severe TS have said that they would rather be dead than cope with the 'twitches' for ever.

However, other individuals cope by treating their disorder with fondness. Some individuals call it 'my syndrome' and find this comforting. An adult patient of ours calls it her 'G & T'. A young girl patient of ours calls her coprolalia 'Ethel'. Others give their obsessive–compulsive disorder or tics a variety of other names, which helps the individual have, in a way, two personas—one with TS and one without.

Talking about the problems to friends and relatives

In addition to telling siblings, parents will also have to let their own parents and families know that their child has TS. It is as well to bear in mind that the news may be distressing for grandparents, although they may feel uneasy about sharing their distress. One particular area that some families feel sensitive about, and that can cause difficulty, concerns the possible hereditary factors involved in the syndrome (see also Chapter 10). It is important in this respect for families to be aware of the relevant information while not getting caught up in unhelpful recriminations such as 'It's not on our side of the family'.

The issues are complex and other close relatives planning a family may find it helpful to seek the advice of an expert in genetic counselling. We know of one case where, after hearing that TS is genetic, a mother requested a termination of her next pregnancy, which was granted. Unfortunately, in this case no clear genetic counselling was sought, which might have made the couple consider their choices in the light of all the information available. Had she discussed it with appropriate professionals in more detail, she might not have chosen to have the termination. Several parents ask us if they should have another child. The answer is clear 'Yes, if you would like another'. Remember that people with TS can be ordinary or highly successful (see Chapter 13).

Much the same advice as that for talking to relatives also holds when dealing with friends and acquaintances—it is important to provide open and straightforward information about the child's TS 'disorder'. This is the most effective way of preventing misunderstandings caused by ignorance or prejudice. However, it can be easier said than done. It can sometimes be quite challenging to think of ways of dealing with the critical looks or comments that parents may get when their child behaves strangely in public, such as swearing inappropriately and out of the blue, or being hyperactive and constantly running about and climbing on to things. Other parents of children with TS may often have useful advice on how to tackle these sorts of problems. An example of an introductory card is given in Appendix 1.

We often recommend that parents and patients join their national TS Association (in the UK this has now been renamed Tourettes Action) or Foundation and thus find support from parents and individuals who have similar problems. Judgement needs to be exercised of course. For example, if the child is an uncomplicated case, parents do not always do well by contacting parents whose children have much more complex problems. We usually discuss the pros and cons of joining the association, tailoring the discussion to the individuals concerned. In the UK, Tourettes Action has a telephone helpline that serves families during the working week. Tourettes Action (in the UK), TS Associations in the USA, the Canadian TS Foundation, and others also have 'question and answer' information leaflets. These are professional and authoritative, and some people with TS carry these leaflets with them, ready to offer them to those who ask awkward questions! These organizations also have local area groups (chapters) that run meetings and support groups. Joining an organization such as Tourettes Action (UK), the TS Association, or TS Foundation can lead to discovering lots of practical tips, such as names of hotels that have an understanding and progressive policy towards people with disabilities, making holidays that much easier. They can also give advice on benefits and other entitlements. By making contact with other individuals in the same situation, one can learn how they are coping and, in that way, feel less isolated or overwhelmed by one's own situation. Some parents even begin to believe that, with others, they can work to make the world a better place not only for their own child, but for all children and individuals with TS.

Immediate consequences of diagnosis

◆   If you or your child's condition fits the clinical picture of TS, at first it may seem that your worst fears have come true. Secretly you may have been hoping to hear that the problems were only mild and would pass. The diagnosis may then be a shock. However, there are many different reactions and many different stages in the reaction to the diagnosis of TS.

◆ Many of the children who are diagnosed are unaware of the implications of diagnosis and thus are largely unaffected by receiving it. Parents and adult patients differ widely in their reactions to the diagnosis.

◆ Whatever the response, parents and patients often feel apprehension about the future and confusion about the condition. Receipt of a confirmed TS diagnosis should be followed up by sensitive discussion with the family (parents, carers, spouse, partner) about the nature of the problems, their severity, and the expected future course. Further information and support should always be provided.

9

Is there more than one type of Tourette syndrome?

➜ Key points

- The original description of TS included multiple tics, coprolalia, and echolalia.

- According to current diagnostic criteria, TS is a unitary condition.

- Clinical observations suggest that there is more than one type of TS.

- Community and clinical studies show that 90 per cent of patients with TS have other problems.

- Recent statistical studies agree that there is at least one specific type of TS. About 10 per cent of all patients with TS have this type, *i.e. pure simple motor and vocal tics*. This has been replicated several times.

- Studies also suggest that another type of TS may include complex tics.

- Studies also suggest that a further type of TS may include aggressive and/or socially inappropriate behaviours.

◆ Other phenotypes, types, or factors may include alone or in combination:

compulsions

coprophenomena, echophenomena, paliphenomena

attention deficit–hyperactivity disorder (ADHD)

obsessive–compulsive disorder

anxiety, depression, obsessionality, and self–injurious behaviours.

A historical perspective

We have already shown that calculating the prevalence of TS (i.e. the number of subjects having TS at a certain time) is more complex than was once thought. Until fairly recently TS was thought to be a rare and, according to some, a psychogenically mediated bizarre curiosity. Prevalence depends, at least in part, on the definition of TS. The internationally accepted diagnostic criteria demand that a person must have both motor and vocal (phonic) tics for longer than a year to obtain the diagnosis of TS. We have shown that prevalence figures for TS vary between 0.4 and 3.8 per cent for youngsters between the ages of 5 and 18 years. It has been calculated that of over 400 000 young people studied internationally, 1 per cent were diagnosed as having TS (see Chapter 3).

When Georges Gilles de la Tourette first described TS in 1885 he emphasized the triad of multiple motor tics, coprolalia, and echolalia. Thereafter all internationally accepted diagnostic criteria have stipulated that TS is a *unitary single condition* and that the presence of multiple motor and one or more vocal (phonic) tics for over a year is sufficient to make a diagnosis of TS. However, those in clinical practice observed that there were many types of patients, and a pragmatic classification based on these observations was as follows: 'simple TS' (simple motor and vocal tics only), 'full-blown TS' (tics together with coprolalia, echolalia, and palilalia), and 'TS plus' (tics together with comorbid conditions or psychopathology, which we have discussed before). Thereafter several studies in both epidemiological or community settings as well as in dedicated TS clinics showed that about 90 per cent of patients with TS also have comorbid conditions. The other side of the coin is that only 10 per cent of patients with TS do not have these other conditions and have only tics.

Genotype versus phenotype

Let us examine the phenotype and genotype. A genotype is an individual's genetic make-up. The presence of a gene means that a person will inherit a particular characteristic from their parents, and therefore certain diseases and features are hereditary. If a person has the specific gene for Huntington's disease, they will eventually get Huntington's disease, and this will be in the person's 'genetic make-up' even long before the person gets the actual disease. Thus the *genotype cannot* be 'seen' by the naked eye, but can be tested for by blood tests. The genotype can be tested early on in life, although different countries have different rules about allowing genetic testing in young people. Another 'genotype' is a disorder called 'trisomy 21', which is caused by an incorrect number of chromosomes—there are too many (three instead of two) chromosomes 21. This is the genetic make-up of Down syndrome.

The *phenotype* is what we *can* see with the naked eye in a person. For instance, the phenotype of Huntington's disease may include chorea-like movements and eventually dementia. However, these occur only when the person is older. The phenotype of Down syndrome is what one sees with the naked eye—a person with the characteristic features of Down syndrome.

Genotype and phenotype in TS

In TS the cause is largely genetic, but as yet there is no genetic test, no blood test, and no clear genotype. Therefore we have to rely entirely on the phenotype, i.e. what doctors and other people can see or observe in a patient. This is how doctors currently make the diagnosis of TS. We take a history and examine the patient with TS (see Chapter 4). However, there are some problems with the diagnosis of TS. The division of motor and phonic tics may be slightly arbitrary; for example, sniffing is certainly a sound. It was once thought to be a motor tic but 'evolved' to become a vocal or phonic tic. It could be argued that only tics that actually arise from the vocal cords, such as sounds including coprophenomena, echophenomena, and actual words, are truly vocal tics. Throat-clearing, coughing, and gulping are probably somewhere in the middle but are now always considered as vocal or phonic tics. It is for that reason that 'sound' tics are often currently referred to as phonic rather than vocal, so as not to imply involvement of the vocal cords.

Recent research into the TS phenotype

Recent research data using sophisticated statistical tests such as cluster analysis and factor analysis agree with these clinical observations and suggest that

TS is *not* a unitary (single) condition, thereby raising a challenge to the currently accepted international diagnostic criteria. The research has shown that there may well be different types of TS. The prevalence of TS in these individual subtypes is unknown.

Since Itard documented the case of the famous Marquise de Dampierre in 1825 and Gilles de la Tourette described the disorder in 1885, when he emphasized the triad of motor tics, coprolalia, and echolalia, the various definitions of TS in the American DSM Classification, such as the age at onset and the presence of distress, have changed. Also, the swearing tic or coprolalia has never been required for diagnosis in any of the diagnostic schedules. However, both the DSM (American) and ICD (World Health Organization) criteria have always suggested, and indeed stipulated, that TS is a *unitary condition, i.e. that is there is only one type*. But the causes of TS are complex and there is highly likely to be more than one gene and therefore more than one genotype. There are also other causes that contribute to TS, which are not genetic.

What is also difficult is that the recent studies we have outlined have suggested that there is also more than one phenotype. Only a few studies have tried to classify patients with TS on the basis of their tic phenomenology. The effects of psychopathology should be taken into account when considering phenotype and, therefore, prevalence (how common) and epidemiology (where TS occurs). Early studies examined the phenotype or clinical symptoms of patients with TS, describing the full extent of the associated clinical phenomenology (symptoms) and psychopathology (psychiatric problems), and in the 1980s our group demonstrated significant associations between various 'core' features of TS, such as the fact that aggression, hostility, and obsessionality were significantly associated with copro- and echophenomena as well as with a family history of tics or TS.

In addition, although not directly comparable, all studies to date using cluster or factor analysis have shown two or more factors, i.e. two or more phenotypes. In all studies that have specifically examined for it, one factor has included simple motor and phonic/vocal tics. Thus, it can be concluded that the TS phenotype is *heterogeneous* and not unitary as suggested by both the DSM and ICD criteria, and also that one phenotype may well consist of 'simple motor and phonic tics only'. Only a few studies have been published to date (Dr Pauls and Dr Mathews in America, and our group). Thus the phenotype of TS is much more complicated than was previously thought and there is almost certainly clinical heterogeneity. In other words, there are probably many types of TS in both clinic and community settings. These differing phenotypes would certainly affect calculations of TS prevalence.

Whether or not the various phenotypes are associated with different causes has not been widely studied, and the few such studies examining phenotypic manifestations in the light of presumed causative factors are summarized here. One study showed that three of the four factors that they identified were heritable (genetic). Another study examined phenotypic features of ABGA-positive and ABGA-negative TS children and adults (ABGA is the acronym for anti-basal ganglia antibodies, a marker of autoimmunity following strepto-coccus infections, which has been related to TS (see Chapter 10)). On statistical testing, ADHD was inversely correlated with ABGA, i.e. those who had ADHD did not have ABGA. Lastly, a twin study showed that among twins who were concordant for tic diagnosis (i.e. both twins had tics) but not for severity, those with more severe tics had lower birth-weights. Thus it seems that various causes may well be associated with various phenotypes, but further studies are required before any conclusions can be drawn.

In conclusion, recent studies suggest that there is more than one TS phenotype, and the type that has been replicated in every study is simple motor and vocal (phonic) tics. In the majority of individuals these tics will be mild, and will probably go unnoticed by the individual and his/her family, friends, and colleagues.

❌ Myths about TS

- All people with TS are the same.

- All people with TS have coprolalia (swearing tic).

- All people with TS have socially inappropriate behaviours.

- There is only one type of TS.

- All people with TS are severely affected.

10

What causes Tourette Syndrome?

> **Key points**

The cause of TS was unknown for a long time, and indeed the precise areas and circuits within the brain are still not completely identified. However, it is clear that the cause of TS is complex and is made up of:

- genetic influences in the vast majority of cases, but no single gene has been convincingly identified

- certain infections in a subgroup of patients

- pregnancy and birth difficulties in some patients

- possibly hormonal influences.

Is there a biochemical cause of TS?

The absolute neurochemical basis for TS is, as yet, unknown. However, the main biochemical theory is that there is an imbalance in the function of a neurotransmitter (a messenger in the brain) called *dopamine*. This theory is based mainly on the beneficial effect of dopamine-blocking drugs, and on the fact that certain stimulants, such as pemoline and methylphenidate, can cause tics to worsen.

However, a number of studies have found other neurochemical abnormalities. For example, patients with TS seem to have lower levels of *serotonin*, another neurotransmitter, which concentrates in areas of the brain called the subthalamus and the basal ganglia. There also seems to be a reduction in cyclic-AMP (another chemical messenger in the brain). Other abnormalities that have been found include alterations in the noradrenergic system and an increased number of dopamine uptake carrier sites in the striatum of the brain. In a few cases a decrease in dynorphin (a naturally occurring opioid-like substance) has been demonstrated in the globus pallidus (part of the basal ganglia). Finally, abnormalities of the opioid system have been found in the frontal areas of the brain.

Does electrophysiology reveal any abnormalities?

Electroencephalographic (EEG) testing measures electrical activity in the brain. Studies show that EEG patterns in patients with TS are mostly normal, and if abnormalities are found, they are minor and non-specific and not related to the actual tics. There is also no specific relationship between epilepsy and TS.

Have researchers been able to pinpoint the affected areas of the brain?

So far there have been very few post-mortem studies of the brain tissue of people with TS. Those that have been reported show abnormalities in the caudate nucleus within the basal ganglia (an area of the brain concerned with movement) and the anterior cingulate cortex, and their connections with the periaqueductal grey matter and midbrain tegmentum.

What does neuroimaging (brain scanning) reveal?

Neuroimaging has revolutionized the way we study the brain, but in TS these techniques are used mainly in research, rather than in routine everyday clinical practice. Two aspects of the brain may be studied.

Structural brain studies

Computed tomography (CT) scans of the brain have not revealed any abnormalities that might throw light on the cause of TS. A few cases of abnormal CT scans have been documented in the medical literature, but by far the majority have been normal. *Magnetic resonance imaging* (MRI) scans of the structure of the brain have been able to detect more subtle abnormalities than have CT scans. Fairly consistent abnormalities that have been reported by several groups include abnormalities of the size of the caudate nucleus (part of the basal ganglia). One large study showed that caudate nucleus volumes were significantly smaller in both children and adults with TS. The lenticular nucleus volumes were also smaller in adults and children with TS who were diagnosed as having comorbid obsessive–compulsive disorder (OCD).

These volume differences did not correlate significantly with the severity of the tic, OCD, or attention deficit–hyperactivity disorder symptoms. Dr Peterson, the author, suggested that reduced caudate nucleus volumes may be a good 'candidate marker' for a trait (long-standing) abnormality in the structure of the basal ganglia in persons with TS. Smaller lenticular nucleus volumes may be an additional marker for the presence of comorbid OCD and for the persistence of tic symptoms into adulthood. Abnormalities have also been demonstrated in the size of the corpus callosum (which divides and transfers information across the two halves of the brain), as well as the symmetry of other basal ganglia structures, the size of the lateral ventricles, and loss of normal ventricular asymmetry.

Functional brain studies

Functional imaging of the brain using *positron emission tomography* (PET) has found metabolic and blood flow abnormalities in the basal ganglia, as well as in the fronto-temporal areas, especially in the putamen. In a PET study undertaken by our group, it was demonstrated that simple motor tics were associated with a part of the brain called the sensorimotor cortex, while more complex tics (such as coprolalia and clear vocal tics) were shown to be associated with activity in other parts of the brain called the pre-rolandic and post-rolandic language regions, as well as in other areas including the insula, caudate, thalamus, and cerebellum. These data are quite exciting as they suggest that different types of tics may indeed have different underlying biological mechanisms. Studies examining cerebral blood flow using *single-photon emission computed tomography* (SPECT) have found lower levels of blood flow in the basal ganglia, thalamus, and frontal and temporal cortical areas, as well as elevated frontal cortex blood flow (relative to the basal ganglia, and again including the caudate nucleus and putamen).

Summary

Both functional and subtle structural abnormalities appear to be present in the brains of people with TS, especially in the *fronto-temporal areas* and the *basal ganglia* when compared with groups of healthy controls.

Are genetic factors involved in causing TS?

There is no doubt that genetic factors are involved in TS in the majority of cases, but the precise mechanisms of inheritance are unknown. A few sporadic cases of TS do occur and these must be due to acquired abnormalities in the brain, such as in the basal ganglia.

To date, the genetic basis of TS has not been discovered and there is no blood test for the disorder (see Chapter 4). Therefore we shall discuss some of the main genetic hypotheses advanced so far.

Four ways in which TS might be passed down in families and thus inherited have been suggested. These genetic models are:

(1) autosomal dominant

(2) mixed model

(3) polygenic model

(4) bilinear inheritance.

Most support to date has been for *autosomal dominant* inheritance. This means that if an individual has TS, there is a 50–50 chance that each offspring will inherit the gene. However, there has been a suggestion of *incomplete penetrance*. This means that even if an individual carries the gene, it is not 100 per cent certain that he/she will display the symptoms. This type of inheritance suggests the presence of a *single major gene*. It has also been suggested that obsessive–compulsive behaviour may be one of the symptoms (or part of the phenotype) caused by the gene. That is, if an individual inherits the gene, he/she might display obsessive–compulsive behaviour instead of, or as well as, TS.

The *mixed model* suggests there is one major gene that does not behave strictly according to classic (Mendelian) laws; it is intermediate between recessive (requiring two genes) and dominant (only requiring one gene to be manifest). In this model it is suggested that there is a genetic predisposition involving one copy of the gene that renders an individual vulnerable, and other factors (such as infections, or factors in pregnancy or at birth) that determine the extent of the expression of the gene. The number of genes (one or two) may, in turn, determine the severity of the disorder in any given individual.

The *polygenic model* is currently somewhat controversial. In this model, multiple genes are involved and no single gene exerts a major effect. It is proposed that there is a threshold number of several genes required to produce TS within a given individual.

In *bilinear* inheritance, an individual inherits the genetic vulnerability from both the maternal and paternal sides.

To complicate matters yet further, it has recently been suggested that there may be *genetic heterogeneity*, i.e. different genes may be responsible for TS in different families.

The majority of chromosomes in patients with TS are normal. Chromosomes are composed of many genes, which are blueprints for making the proteins that are the building blocks of life. The search for the TS gene(s) is currently taking place around the world. There is also a USA TSA International Genetic Research Consortium of several centres in the USA, Canada, the UK (including Professor Mary Robertson), Canada, South Africa and The Netherlands investigating the genetic cause of TS.

Recently, dopamine receptor D2 genes were shown to be associated with TS in some individuals. Five complete genome scans in TS have been reported, and the regions of interest have been shown to be on chromosomes 2, 4, 5, 7, 8, 10, 11, 13, 17, 18, and 19. It has also been suggested that the DRD4 and MAO-A genes may confer an increased risk for developing TS, but no significant linkage results have been obtained and replicated. Currently, most interest is focused on chromosome 2.

In 2005, a group of scientists reported the association of TS with the gene SLITRK1 on chromosome 13q31.1 in a small number of individuals with TS. This is the first indication of an actual gene being involved in some cases of TS. However, other researchers have provided evidence that mutations (changes) in the SLITRK1 gene are probably only a very rare cause of TS, and tests designed to detect variants in the SLITRK1 gene do not have diagnostic utility in clinical practice. The earlier findings published in 2005 in the high-profile journal *Science*, which aroused much medical and media interest, have not been replicated by other researchers.

To date, no genetic linkage studies have been replicated and much of the genome has been excluded, i.e. no particular gene has yet been found to be the actual cause of TS. Thus the genetics of TS are complex and there is almost certainly genetic as well as clinical heterogeneity. In addition, many authorities believe that an individual may inherit a vulnerability to a spectrum disorder, including TS and obsessive–compulsive behaviours, and only a few suggest that attention deficit–hyperactivity disorder may also be included: most agree that TS and ADHD are not genetically related.

Are any other factors involved in causing TS?

Other possible causes for TS include:

◆ infections

◆ birth difficulties

◆ allergy

◆ hormones

◆ stress.

It should be noted that the aetiology (cause) of TS was originally considered to be psychological, and indeed even psychoanalytical, but over the last few years large families have been documented with many related people affected by TS, tics, or obsessive–compulsive symptomatology, suggesting a familial nature. However, as we have seen, no actual gene has been identified and replicated as being *causal* in TS. Therefore other aetiologies or causes have also been investigated.

Infections

There have been some recent studies suggesting that the body's autoimmune mechanisms may play a role in the onset or exacerbation of TS or obsessive symptoms. Neuroimmunological theories operating via the process of molecular mimicry have become of interest in the TS field over the last decade. In the late nineteen-nineties a group of researchers described a group of 50 children with OCD and tic disorders, designated as *paediatric autoimmune neuropsychiatric disorders associated with streptococcal infections*, or PANDAS. The best evidence for a relationship between TS and streptococcal infections (e.g. recurrent sore throats, tonsillitis, etc.) comes from a study where the authors found that patients with TS, OCD, or tic disorder were more likely than healthy people (controls) to have had prior streptococcal infection in the 3 months before the date of onset. A few other controlled studies have found laboratory evidence of group A beta-haemolytic streptococcus (GABHS) infections and/or increased levels of antibodies reacting against basal ganglia antibodies (antibasal ganglia antibodies (ABGAs)) in some patients with TS, supporting a role of streptococcal infection and basal ganglia autoimmunity in TS, but other groups have failed to confirm these findings. It seems unlikely that GABHS infections directly cause TS, but it may well be that individuals inherit a *susceptibility to TS* and also inherit *the way they react* to some infections. Thus, most authors, including our own group and collaborators, suggest that there is an association between streptococcal infections and TS in a subgroup of patients.

Birth factors

An American, Dr Leckman, first suggested that birth factors play a role in the development of TS and outlined the potential role of pre- and perinatal (before and around birth) events in the pathogenesis of TS. He suggested that the mothers of children with tics were more likely to have experienced a complication during pregnancy than the mothers of children who did not have tics, that the severity of maternal life stress during pregnancy (including severe nausea and/or vomiting during the first trimester) are risk factors for developing tic disorders, and that premature low-birthweight children, as well as those with low Apgar scores and more frequent maternal prenatal visits, were associated with having TS. A rigorous subsequent study by Dr Burd involving 92 cases with TS and 460 matched controls identified four variables in the TS children (first trimester prenatal care initiated, Apgar score at 5 minutes, first month prenatal care begun, and number of prenatal visits) as potential risk factors for the development of TS. Thus, in conclusion and in general, it appears that people with TS often have pregnancy and birth-related issues.

Allergy

It has been reported that tics can worsen with seasonal allergies, or when allergens in food are eaten. Drugs used to treat allergies may also increase tics. Although there may be food intolerance in some patients, to date there is little scientific evidence of the involvement of allergy in TS. Individual patients may be allergic to certain substances (e.g. chocolate), and of course they are advised to avoid these foods. People with TS are affected by allergies in no greater number than the general population. However, if an individual patient's tics become worse after having, say, chocolate, caffeine, or Coca Cola, then it is best for that particular person not to have the 'three Cs', but clearly this does not apply to all people with TS.

Hormones and stress

Finally, clinical experience and some medical research suggests an association between stressful life events and fluctuations in symptom severity of patients with tic disorder while Leckman and his group have also raised the hypothesis that androgen exposure ('prenatal masculinization of the brain') may also be important in the aetiopathogenesis (cause and development) of TS and tic-related disorders.

Conclusions

In conclusion, the causes of TS are much more complex than previously recognized. A number of factors may be important in determining just how the symptoms of TS are expressed, with complex genetic mechanisms, some infections, and pre- and perinatal difficulties also affecting the clinical presentation of TS. These all probably interact to produce the very special profile of symptoms and severity that is unique to each person with TS.

11

Which therapies are most useful for Tourette syndrome?

⊅ Key points

◆ Management includes reassurance, explanation, and psychoeducation about TS.

◆ Behaviour therapies such as habit reversal training are superior to psychotherapy for tics.

◆ Cognitive-behavioural therapy is helpful for obsessive–compulsive behaviour (OCB)/obsessive–compulsive disorder.

◆ Medications such as the typical and atypical (newer and better tolerated) neuroleptics remain the mainstay of the treatment of the tics.

◆ Other medications can be used for attention deficit–hyperactivity disorder (ADHD), OCB/OCD, and depression.

◆ A recent novel, but rare, treatment by experts for adults with severe TS who have not responded to other treatments is deep brain stimulation.

Which therapies are most useful for patients with TS?

Both counselling and medication have proved useful in treating people with TS. *Explanation and reassurance* may be sufficient for many adult patients with a mild form of the condition. Similarly, parents of mildly affected children may feel that the diagnosis and an explanation about the nature of TS, plus information about self-help groups and booklets for teachers, are sufficient. The management for severely affected patients, who may have the associated features of OCB, ADHD, self-injury, or aggressive behaviour, is more complex.

♦ Individual psychotherapy is useful for reducing and coping with the daily difficulties of living with tics, but the tics themselves are not responsive to psychotherapy and therefore should not be the target of treatment.

♦ Behaviour therapies, including massed negative practice, relaxation training, and contingency management, have been used in TS. The technique most frequently used has been *massed negative practice* (over-rehearsal of the target tic, such as excessive blinking) in which the patient performs the movement for a specified time, interspersed with periods of rest. It is suggested to the patient that he/she becomes tired of doing the tic, resulting in a decrease in its frequency. This method does show some therapeutic benefit in TS.

♦ *Contingency management* holds that behaviours are maintained by the consequences that follow them. Therefore patients are positively reinforced (for example, by praise) for not performing tics or performing alternative behaviours. This has been used with some success, mainly on children. This method is usually used in combination with other behavioural methods.

♦ *Relaxation training* has also been used in combination with other methods and includes, for example, muscular tensing and relaxing and deep breathing. This may help to reduce the tics for a short period of time.

♦ *Habit reversal training* is a promising behavioural technique for treating TS. In a nutshell, it works by increasing the subject's awareness of the tic and developing an appropriate competing response, so that the muscles used for the new action make it impossible to perform the actual tic. For example, instead of eye-blinking, the patient would be taught and encouraged by the therapist to gently close his/her eyelids and hold them closed for a few seconds.

In summary, behaviour therapy plays an important role in the effective management of TS, especially in patients with a simple motor or vocal tic and OCB. It may be useful as an adjunct to medication, or may be used alone in patients who are not responding to any treatments, or who experience unwanted side effects of medication.

Which medications are recommended?

To date there is no cure for TS, but there are many medications that successfully reduce the various manifestations.

At present, medication is the main treatment for the motor and vocal tics, as well as some of the associated behaviours of TS. The medications most commonly used are neuroleptics, antipsychotics, or dopamine antagonists. These are divided into the older 'typical' drugs and the newer 'atypical' drugs, which differ primarily in their side-effect profiles. These medications are also called *major tranquillizers*, not because they tranquillize people (especially not people with TS, as they are given relatively small doses), but as a way of differentiating them from the minor tranquillizers or anxiolytics (mainly the benzodiazepine family of drugs (diazepam/Valium)). Another reason for the distinction is that, in higher doses, the neuroleptics are administered for traditionally major psychiatric illnesses (such as mania or schizophrenia), whereas the anxiolytics are given for traditionally relatively 'minor' ailments (such as anxiety and sleep disturbance).

Double-blind trials have been undertaken and published for several of the older or *'typical' antipsychotics*, such as haloperidol, pimozide, sulpiride, and tiapride, and have shown that the medications are superior to placebo in reducing tics. In lay terms, a double-blind trial means that the active ingredient (medication) is tested against an inactive agent ('sugar pill') that looks the same. Throughout the study neither the patients nor the researchers knows which patient is taking what agent until the 'code' is broken afterwards. This is the gold standard of all research studies. However, few experts today use the older atypicals as first-line agents because of unacceptable side effects.

As sulpiride and tiapride are different from the other drugs, some doctors regard them as being halfway between the typicals and the atypicals. Many experts in the UK use sulpiride as their first-line agent because it is recommended in the *British National Formulary* and does not have the side effects of the older drugs.

Newer neuroleptics (also called *atypical antipsychotics*), namely risperidone, aripiprazole (which is actually a dopamine partial agonist), quetiapine, and ziprasidone, have recently been added to the pharmacological armamentarium. Risperidone is the only one of these that has been shown to work in double-blind trials. Preliminary studies of the others have shown promising results consisting of significant efficacy coupled with better tolerability. Ziprasidone is not available in the UK. Several of these medications, such as aripiprazole, are available in a liquid preparation, which is easier for many individuals, especially children, to take.

Clonidine (often also used in the treatment of headaches, migraine, and hypertension or high blood pressure) has also been used with some success to reduce the tics in TS. It is especially recommended if a child has TS and associated ADHD. It can also be prescribed as a transdermal patch on the skin. Clonidine has side effects and may be associated with tiredness or depression. It must *never* be stopped suddenly, as this can result in a dangerous rise in blood pressure ('rebound hypertension'). Recently, a drug similar to clonidine called *guanfacine* has also been shown to be useful, and may well have fewer side effects than clonidine, but it is not available in the UK. Other medications for the ADHD symptoms include the *stimulants*, methylphenidate and pemoline, as well as the *tricyclic antidepressants*, desipramine and imipramine. Methylphenidate is available as a short-acting prepation (Ritalin) and as once-daily sustained release preparation (Concerta or Equasym).

Finally, the relatively new *selective serotonin-reuptake inhibitors* (SSRIs) (e.g. fluoxetine, fluvoxamine, sertraline, paroxetine, citalopram, and escitalopram) can be used to treat the OCB aspects of the syndrome, as well as when the patient is depressed. SSRIs can also be helpful with impulse control difficulties. However, the doses are different, being higher (e.g. fluoxetine 60 mg daily) for the obsessive–compulsive aspects of TS and lower (e.g. fluoxetine 20 mg daily) for depression. In the UK there are strict guidelines as to which of these can be prescribed to young people, and the only one actually allowed is fluoxetine. The concern is that suicidal ideas and behaviours have been reported with SSRIs, and extra care should be taken with young people who may act (on the suicide idea) before telling anyone.

The older tricyclic antidepressant *clomipramine*, which also acts on serotonin, is useful for the obsessive–compulsive aspects and depression. The many side effects of clomipramine and the fact that it is dangerous in overdose, make it less acceptable to many clinicians. Recently, *tetrabenazine* has also been documented as useful in reducing symptoms of TS. Tetrabenazine is usually prescribed by neurologists and has been associated with depression.

Newer pharmacological strategies have been tried with some success, but to date only with relatively small numbers of patients. These include nicotine transdermal patches (worn on the skin), calcium-channel blockers, and injections of botulinum toxin into localized areas (e.g. for excessive eye blinking, also known as blepharospasm).

Most common medications for tics

Dopamine-modulating drugs (neuroleptics)

- Typical antipsychotics

  Haloperidol

  Pimozide

- Substituted benzamides

  Sulpiride

  Tiapride

- (Newer) atypical antipsychotics

  Risperidone

  Ziprasidone

  Aripiprazole

  Quetiapine

Other drugs

- Clonidine

- Guanfacine

- Tetrabenazine

What are the side effects of these medications?

Side effects, such as dystonia or stiffness, rigidity, and tremor, as well as sedation and depression are common with haloperidol, but are less common with pimozide. The neuroleptics may also cause concentration problems, cognitive blunting, and, rarely, tardive dyskinesia (a movement disorder that consists of lip, mouth, and tongue movements). Sulpiride has fewer side effects of this sort (i.e. fewer extrapyramidal problems) as well as fewer sedative side effects, although gynaecomastia (enlargement of the breasts in men), galactorrhoea (excessive unnatural production of milk by the breasts), menstrual irregularities, and depression have been reported.

With the neuroleptics, these side effects can be avoided by starting with a small dose (e.g. a haloperidol dose of 0.5 mg daily) and increasing it by 0.5 mg every week until a point is reached with maximum benefit and minimum side effects. Reports about changes in electrocardiogram (ECG; heart beat) patterns with pimozide have, naturally, raised some concern, and so it is important that patients have a baseline (before treatment) ECG to rule out any heart problems. If the patient has the heart condition called the long QT syndrome, pimozide should not be used. If there are other heart problems, the patient should have routine ECGs under the guidance of a cardiologist. Prescribing neuroleptics to children with TS may also be useful, but again there are reports of side effects and therefore careful monitoring is required.

Currently, the most frequently prescribed medications for TS are probably the recently introduced *atypical antipsychotics*, which are characterized by a *significantly improved tolerability profile*. These medications (especially risperidone, and the newer aripiprazole) seem to combine good efficacy with acceptable manageability; the most commonly reported side effects are restlessness, daytime sleepiness, and gastrointestinal (e.g. nausea) and sleep disturbances.

Clonidine has fewer and milder side effects than the neuroleptics in general, with the most common being sedation. Sedation occurs in about 10–20 per cent of cases and is dose related; tolerance often develops with time. Other side effects include insomnia, nocturnal restlessness, dry mouth, headaches, dizziness, postural hypotension (lowering of blood pressure especially when standing up), and, occasionally, rashes. The tricyclics can cause dry mouth, constipation, blurring of vision, and dizziness. The SSRIs can cause gastric upset, such as nausea. Methylphenidate and pemoline, which are stimulants, can cause loss of appetite and weight, initial insomnia (difficulty in falling asleep), gastrointestinal upset (e.g. nausea), and headaches.

Tetrabenazine has also been used with success in TS. It reduces pre-synaptic (before the nerve ending) monoamines, and blocks post-synaptic (after the nerve ending) dopamine receptors. The main advantage of tetrabenazine is that it rarely causes side effects such as dystonia (acute stiffness) or tardive dyskinesia (mouth movements that occur after long-term high dosage of standard neuroleptics). Side effects that do occur include drowsiness, fatigue, depression, sleeping difficulties, and a feeling of foot/leg restlessness.

Neurosurgery

Neurosurgery is *not*, and we repeat *not*, often used in people with TS. Our group did undertake neurosurgery in the 1990s in patients who were extremely severely affected and resistant to all treatments. Few doctors today perform traditional *ablative* (*destructive*) structural surgery for TS.

However, a relatively rarely used and novel *non-ablative reversible functional* type of neurosurgery called deep brain stimulation (DBS) has recently been used successfully in many other movement disorders, such as Parkinson's disease, tremor, and dystonia, and also in depression. DBS entails the implantation of stimulating electrodes in the deep structures of the brain that are connected to a machine similar to a heart pacemaker, which keeps the stimulator in action. DBS has relatively recently been reported as successful in a small number of patients (a few dozen) with TS. The main 'targets' for DBS in TS have been the centromedian–parafascicular complex of the thalamus, the internal globus pallidus (part of the basal ganglia), and, more rarely, the internal capsule, but there is still international debate as to which are the best or correct targets. Strict protocols for DBS have been published: it can only be used in centres with experts in both TS and DBS, and it must not generally be done on persons under 25 years of age as TS symptoms usually reduce by the age of 18 years (see Chapter 7). In addition, the patients must be resistant to *all* other types of treatment, including medications and behavioural treatments, and their quality of life must be severely reduced. A Dutch–Flemish group pioneered DBS in TS and an Italian group has performed the most DBS procedures. Although the preliminary reports suggest remarkably good efficacy and safety, the numbers are still small and there are no long-term data on implanted patients with TS.

12

Education, employment, and empowerment

➔ 'E' points

- Education, Education, Education—is for all people—and also for all people with TS.

- Employment and empowerment are important.

- Extra support may be required for some pupils with TS.

- Empathizing with the pupil with TS is important.

- Employment with satisfaction is the hope and reality for most people and also for those with TS.

- Empowerment is important for all people to survive—including those with TS.

- Enable people with TS and they may even Enable you.

- Enclusion (this is a deliberate neologism 'new word')—meaning *include* people with TS.

- Even people with TS can be 'tinkers, tailors, soldiers, sailors', 'rich men, poor men, beggar men' but very few thieves!

These eight 'Es' are important for anyone in life and also especially for people with TS. Other 'Es' follow from these, and it shows that the 'E word', not only the 'F word' (as a tic), is important in the lives of people with TS. It is an important message to state at the outset that a person with TS can be successful, very successful—as can anyone—and many people with TS are good mothers, fathers, shopkeepers, teachers, doctors, lawyers, and high-flying celebrities. However, many people with TS keep their light hidden under a bushel—for fear of stigma. But that is where public education comes in (see at end of section). In the UK, over the years the Government Departments for Education (Department for Education and Employment, Department for Education and Skills, Department for Children, Schools, and Families) have produced guidelines and documents that are available publicly and as such should be consulted when in doubt about any matters relating to the education and employment of anyone—but also those with TS. An Early Day Motion was also signed by 99 Members of Parliament in 2006 (see end of chapter)—all this helps the person and family with TS in their worlds.

Education

Education for the person with TS

How common are tics and TS in school children?

Motor tics occur in about 7–28 per cent of school-aged children. However, as we said in Chapter 3, the accepted prevalence of TS (i.e. how common TS is) is about 1 per cent of youngsters in mainstream schools and in the community. It is unclear what proportion of children who have tics actually have TS, or indeed have one of the other tic disorders, such as chronic multiple tic disorder (CMT) or transient tic disorder (TTD). It should be noted that prevalence figures have been calculated from worldwide studies, but may well be under-estimates as many individuals with TS in certain populations may be unrecognized. Even in special populations (e.g. special schools which usually focus on a disproportionate number of severe or complex cases), students, learners, or pupils with TS may be missed, i.e. the mild cases may be overlooked because they do not come to medical attention. We will use the terms learners, pupils, or students throughout the rest of the chapter.

As we have stated in earlier chapters, in addition to tics, TS can be associated with symptoms such as coprophenomena (uttering obscene words or making obscene gestures), echophenomena (copying behaviours), or behavioural disturbances such as self-injury, obsessive–compulsive behaviour (OCB), and attention deficit–hyperactivity disorder (ADHD). Taken together, this spectrum of clinical problems commonly contributes to school problems in children with TS. This may, in turn, affect their education.

All published studies to date have indicated that the majority of youngsters with TS in schools also experience behavioural difficulties, learning problems including learning disability, mental retardation, needing to repeat a grade, poor grades, and referral to child mental health services. Some require a Statement of Special Educational Needs (SEN) and, as a result, may need special assistance.

For example, in one community-based study using direct clinical examination in the USA, a group of researchers found that 26 per cent of the special education population had definite or probable tics compared with 6 per cent of regular or mainstream classroom students. We have conducted several similar investigations in both mainstream and special schools in the UK examining children for tics and TS, and have found many more tic and TS cases than expected, especially in children with educational problems and autistic spectrum disorders (ASDs). Taken together, these figures suggest that not only is TS in children more common than was once thought (at least 1 per cent), but that it may also be over-represented in special education populations.

What problems do students with TS have at school?

Children with TS may have difficulties in education for a variety of reasons, including the tics themselves, specific learning difficulties, the associated behaviours of obsessive–compulsive behaviours (OCB), obsessive–compulsive disorder, ADHD, oppositional defiant disorder (ODD), conduct disorder (CD), ASD, and/or the side effects of medications (see Chapters 6 and 11).

It must be restated once again that, in our opinion, the majority of mild cases of TS are probably unknown to health professionals, and are well-adjusted people living in the community. To date, no studies have been conducted on the educational profiles of such people. They may have subtle difficulties in learning that do not affect their overall performance and therefore they need no extra help with their education. We have diagnosed TS in adults who have become doctors, lawyers, accountants, teachers, and armed forces personnel. In fact, aspects of TS (e.g. obsessionality) may actually be a strength, not a disability, for people working in all sorts of professions. For example, an obsessional accountant may be known as meticulous and careful. Any of us would surely want to consult such a person.

Some students with TS may encounter problems at school. First, some tics, such as severe head-shaking, neck-stretching, or eye-rolling, may render the child unable to look straight at the teacher for a continuous length of time, or render them unable to read easily, and this can obviously cause educational problems. Similarly, hand tics may interfere with writing, making it untidy or even illegible. Loud and complex vocalizations may interrupt the flow of speech, or disturb the other children in class. Thus the education not only of the pupil with TS, but possibly that of their peers, may also be affected. This, in turn, may have difficult ramifications for the child.

Although studies of children with TS have usually reported the distribution of intelligence (IQ) to be normal, some 'visuospatial deficits' have been documented. These may cause problems such as difficulty in copying things, which children are required to do in a variety of settings (e.g. in homework, or when copying from books or the whiteboard). Children with TS may also have problems with attention and impulsiveness, even if they do not have the full ADHD diagnosis.

However, those TS students who have the associated behaviours of OCB and ADHD will be much more disadvantaged. Youngsters with *obsessions* may become pedantic in their talk and have a need for strict routine, absolute perfection, and having everything 'just right'. This may interfere with a homework assignment, as they may be compelled to do it over and over again, until it is 'just right', at the expense of other assignments that they are unable to do because of lack of sufficient time. We have seen several children who literally take hours to do their homework, far in excess of normal, and often they may never complete it. They may also be slow in their work, because they are always trying to be perfect. Such students may engage in rituals that prevent them from getting on with their schoolwork or homework.

Pupils with both TS and *ADHD* have very special problems. As we stated earlier, ADHD is characterized by poor attention, poor concentration, being easily distracted, fidgeting, hyperactivity, and impulsiveness. Hence, these children often fail to pay close attention to detail, or make careless mistakes in their schoolwork or homework. They often have difficulty in maintaining their attention on schoolwork, or even on enjoyable things such as playing.

Often, the students appear not to be listening when spoken to, and thus they may not actually absorb information, which obviously causes problems. They may also have difficulty in finishing tasks such as schoolwork or homework. They may have special difficulties in organizing things, and may lose things such as toys or their school things (pens, pencils, rubbers (erasers), rulers, books, etc.). They may appear easily distracted, and their work or stream of thought may be interrupted by hearing someone/something outside the classroom, such as in the playground, to whom they may pay more attention than to what is going on in the lesson. This may also cause them to be forgetful and thus not do their homework or other tasks that have been set for them. They may appear to be 'daydreaming' and therefore not paying attention in class.

The *hyperactivity* is also characterized by fidgeting, leaving their desk in the classroom repeatedly, running about, or climbing on things. A hyperactive child in the clinic can cause mayhem—and things can be made worse for the teachers at school by having one or more pupils such as this in a class.

Teachers have a class of about 30 to deal with, and so a child who is hyperactive may cause chaos and needs specific assistance. Children with ADHD may also be noisy, talk too much, or appear always 'on the go'. Their impulsiveness can be demonstrated by their butting into other people's conversations, or answering questions directed at other children in the class.

We see an increasing number of children with TS in the clinic who also have *conduct disorder*. Children with conduct disorder show inappropriate and sometimes severe aggression to people, are cruel to animals, and may, for example, start physical fights in the playground. They may often initiate the bullying of others. They may be very destructive. Some children set fires deliberately, they may lie often and repeatedly, or steal, and might run away from home (even stay out overnight) or play truant from school. Needless to say, these children are especially difficult to deal with at school. Setting boundaries (i.e. saying very clearly what is and what is not acceptable) is important, and they must be reinforced with firm but kind discipline. There is an association between ADHD and conduct disorder, and unfortunately, as mentioned earlier, some of these children grow up to develop what is known as a *personality disorder*. If a child does have these characteristics, it is imperative for the parents to obtain expert advice about management, since otherwise the long-term outlook may not be good. While we see many adult patients with TS with personality disorders in the clinic, in our experience only a few of these end up with serious criminal records. Once again, the incidence of these problems in individuals with mild TS in the community is unknown, but we would not expect it to be high.

In addition to these other medical diagnoses, which can be comorbid (occur) with TS, there are other, often more subtle, problems associated with TS that may also interfere with the youngsters' education. These are called neuropsychological problems, and include executive dysfunction, sensory integration dysfunction, visual–perceptual–motor disabilities, social skills deficits, memory deficits, and 'rage' attacks. These were discussed in more detail in Chapter 6.

Finally, there are also the possible side effects of medication (see Chapter 11), which regrettably may affect learning in students with TS. For example, medications such as sulpiride, haloperidol, pimozide, risperidone, and clonidine may all cause sedation at some level, which might in turn affect the child's concentration. These medications can also cause blurring of vision, which may make reading difficult, although this is not common with the low doses given in TS. There have even been a few reports that some of these medications have caused school phobia and school refusal, but thankfully these are rare. Some medications may also cause depression, which could make a child irritable, 'down', and unwilling to learn. In the UK methylphenidate is sometimes given to pupils with TS who also have ADHD, but it is much more frequently prescribed in the USA and Australia. The prescription of methylphenidate is on the increase in the UK at present. Formerly, only a 'three times a day' preparation was available (with the inherent problems of having to take medication during school hours), but there are now a number of single-dose sustained-release preparations that need only be taken once daily in the morning. Therefore the pupil will have no extra stigma from 'having to take pills' at school (which by definition means that they are 'different' from their peers). Although this medication can reduce the hyperactivity and improve poor concentration, in some individuals it may increase the actual motor and vocal tics, and some children who take it also lose weight.

Students with TS obviously need to be understood. While they may be able to suppress their tics voluntarily, often at the expense of a build-up of inner tension, they do not 'put them on'. The tics are not strictly under voluntary control. Suppression may result in an increase in rebound tics and may cause children social embarrassment. For this reason, attention should not be drawn to the tics. However, teachers should be informed of the tics and behaviours so that they can see the child in terms of his having a recognized disability, rather than being naughty. Unfortunately, we have seen cases of pupils being teased and bullied because of their tics and noises. We believe that some children with TS require special educational assistance (see below).

Working within the context of the National Curriculum

It is important to acknowledge that in Western countries there are educational rules and documents, such as the National Curriculum and the Qualifications and Curriculum Authority (QCA) in the UK. The education of a child with TS must be viewed within the context of the curricula and educational systems, education acts, and rules. Schools and other authorities have to abide by these rules and guidelines, and so it is important to state at the outset that parents, carers, patients, and doctors realize that there is a National Curriculum that most schools choose to follow (independent schools follow other curricula), and consider how best to fit the child with TS into the system chosen. We hope that the following information provides a useful source as well as guidelines as to how this can be achieved.

Finding the correct up-to-date websites and government departments can prove quite difficult, and so we are giving some hints and advice, but acknowledge that some may be slightly out of date, despite our recent searches (March 2008) as departments frequently change names. For example, in the UK many government departments are cited, which at first glance appear quite similar.

'Education' is under the jurisdiction of the Department for Children, Schools, and Families (DCSF), which was formerly known as the Department for Education and Skills (DfES) and the Department for Education and Employment (DfEE). In addition, we have found no single source of information about education, and therefore we have collated and synthesized the main areas and aspects of these departments and educational systems that may affect young people who have TS. We have compiled this from various websites, from discussions with educators, and from a previous book (Carroll and Robertson 2000), and we provide a summary of this below. What follows is our understanding and interpretation of the information, which we hope is as factually correct as possible.

The basic goals that must be incorporated into the education of young people—especially those with TS

Dr Donald Cohen and Dr James Leckman in the USA once stated 'What is critical to later adaptation is the child's sense of himself or herself as competent and loved'. Just how can teachers and educators go about teaching students so that they can learn how to be competent, have self-worth, and have experiences that teach them that they are worthwhile individuals?

Educators and parents can play crucial roles in helping to develop and value the individual, and the basic principles include raising the pupil's self-esteem and self-confidence, helping the building of skills, and acknowledging the pain caused by peer rejection. It is also important to teach skills to build and improve the young person's relationships with other children. Links between poor self-image and low attainment are increasingly being recognized officially in government documents. For example, an old but apt quote suggested that 'Improvements in behaviour are more likely to follow if the child's self-esteem can be enhanced, and if the pupil can be brought to recognize his or her behaviour' (Department for Education 1994). In this respect pupils with TS are no different.

These aims are enshrined in government policy with the Personalized Learning Strategy within 'Every Child Matters Change for Children' programme: 'Change for Children programme is focused on giving every child the support they require, whatever their needs, abilities, background or circumstances. As such, these outcomes tie in closely with the emerging emphasis on personalized learning, which is a key aspect of the new relationship with schools'.

It is important to provide support for pupils when they transfer to different schools, as change is a challenging time for all. Close cooperation between home and school is essential, and should be instigated as soon as possible to plan an easy move. The government has seen this as so important that they have even published 'warning signs', i.e. highlighted those behaviours that may flag up the child most at risk of having difficulty in school or learning environment transition (Department for Children, Schools and Families (DCSF); Department for Education and Skills (DfES)). These 'warning signs' are as follows:

- irregular attendance patterns

- poor social skills and peer relationships

- withdrawn behaviour

- low self-esteem

- difficulties with the curriculum and behavioural problems

- emotional instability.

We have said before that young people with TS integrating or re-integrating from special schools or home tuition into secondary schools or new schools often require extra learning and pastoral support to improve their basic skills before transition.

Parents, carers, and teachers often complain that it is not the tics *per se* that are the most concern with a youngster who has TS, but the 'rages' or tempers that quite a few youngsters with TS have. These rages and tempers in youngsters with TS are well described: there is a sudden 'rage', often in response to, but out of proportion to, a provocation, and afterwards there is often regret and or an apology. However, this can be difficult to handle in a classroom—for the child, for other pupils, and for the teacher. These rages are not well understood medically and are a relatively recently described phenomenon of unsure aetiology (cause). Nevertheless, irrespective of an 'inherent TS-related cause' (such as an abnormality of serotonin, which has been postulated), the child with TS is almost certainly on a 'short fuse' (anger) as a secondary emotion. This secondary emotion may arise from primary emotions, such as fear, frustration, embarrassment, jealousy, and possibly grief, which are linked to having TS. The child sees him/herself as 'different' from what he/she perceives as 'normal children' (those who appear to have no obvious difficulties, have friends, and also do well at school). Therefore it is an important aspect of education to understand and manage this anger, and to help the pupil acquire skills to learn how to handle it.

Equally as important in education, is to teach the child and pupil the importance of forming good relationships—this begins at home with family relationships, and then develops at school with one's peers. It is worth remembering that there are often links between low self-esteem, poor communication abilities, and subsequent disaffection. Many youngsters with TS also have language difficulties and it is important in education to promote language and socialization skills. Many of our patients have been subject to bullying and name calling (e.g. 'nudge nudge wink wink', 'noddy', 'spastic') while at school. There is also an enormous literature on bullying and depression; you will have read in Chapter 6 that both children and adults with TS are particularly prone to depression. In this context it is worth stating that there should be a whole-school approach to bullying. All bullying is unacceptable, and the pupil with TS is probably even more at risk to the 'after-effects' of bullying than more robust 'normal' children. It is worth mentioning at this point that it is not only the tics, noises, ADHD, and rages that may render pupils with TS vulnerable, but they may exhibit involuntary echolalia (copying what other people say) or echopraxia (copying what other people do) and get into trouble for 'taking the mick', which they are not doing on purpose—they cannot help these copying symptoms. The same is important with coprolalia (involuntary swearing)—the pupil with TS may get into trouble or be bullied for 'swearing'.

All schools in the UK have a statutory responsibility to provide pupils with a curriculum for personal, social, and health education (PSHE). PSHE in the National Curriculum is non-statutory, although schools have a responsibility to teach this subject in order to meet their obligations. Much space in the DCSF frameworks for PSHE and Citizenship is devoted to giving schools a basis and guidance on how to deliver these best. The National Healthy School Programme (NHSP) team, based at the Department of Health, together with nine regional coordinators help to build the capacity and capability of local partnerships to support and promote the effective implementation of these frameworks and ideals. We emphasize again that implicit in what we have said is the importance of focusing on positive behaviour, while acknowledging and addressing unacceptable or aggressive behaviours. In addition, all must be aware that there are many ways of encouraging motivation and achievement, and that rewarding pupils helps promote their robust feelings of self-worth; this *obviously* applies to those with TS. Remember that the educator could be teaching a future Dr Samuel Johnson (who compiled the first English Dictionary) or surgeon Mort Doran, or goalkeeper Tim Howard (see Chapter 13). The NHSP produces three main types of publication that may be useful to readers: an e-bulletin, principal NHSP publications, and newsletters.

Other key points to be remembered with respect to the education of pupils with TS is that they may have specific difficulties with mathematics, perfectionism (related to their OCB), daydreaming (ADHD or trying to suppress tics), school phobia (primary or secondary to medication), writing (because of tics), tiredness (many reasons including medication), and poor organizational skills. Finally, improving channels of communication between those involved in the education, health, and upbringing of the child is very important for the education of all children, and particularly those with TS. Specifically, communication between teachers, doctors, nurses, and psychologists and also between the child and the parents or carers is essential for a good educational outcome. All these need to be addressed in full by parents/carers and educators.

What can be achieved?

Most children with TS hope to attain the grades and education that are expected of them. Of course, some do fall behind their peers, especially when they have ADHD, but most actually achieve goals that are acceptable to the young person, their family and teachers. A shining reminder of what can be achieved by individuals with TS is the surgeon Dr Mort Doran (who is also an aeroplane pilot), and the other doctors described in Dr Oliver Sacks' book *An Anthropologist on Mars*), Tim Howard, the famous international goalkeeper, and Peter Hollenbeck, the professor of neuroscience (see Chapter 13). We also have many patients who have attained higher education qualifications and degrees.

Statement of Special Educational Needs (SEN)

In the UK the notion of special needs for certain individuals was enshrined and formalized by the Special Educational Needs and Disability Act 2001 (SENDA). The Disability Discrimination Act 1995 (DDA) was amended in 2005 so that it now gives disabled people rights in the areas of education and other issues (see under Empowerment at the end of this chapter).

In both the UK and many other countries, children with problems require extra support with their studies. In the UK this is supported by a Statement of Special Educational Needs (SEN). This is prepared by an educational psychologist in order to recognize and formalize the provision of special educational help, such as a place in a special school or a personal assistant teacher in a mainstream school. Following an evaluation, the educational psychologist and other professionals involved in the child's care compile a report for the local authority (LA) (formerly called the local education authority (LEA)). This sets the wheels in motion for access to the most suitable school or education for that particular child. When 'statementing' runs smoothly, it is a good way of ensuring the best for a child and keeping the child's needs under review. Parents are invited to comment on and contribute to the draft Statement before it is finalized, so that they should not feel inhibited about expressing their concerns and views.

Much of the information about the SEN is difficult for many to follow as the 'waves' or stages in the procedures, and their names, have changed over the years, but we hope to give an overview and incorporate the information and procedures required. However, it should be remembered that this might well be inaccurate and out of date by the time of publication.

We must also point out that *not all* children who are identified as having special educational needs are given a SEN; in fact, this does not usually happen. Children who are identified by a school as having some kind of special educational need are placed on the school's SEN Register. There are three phases, which are normally termed as wave provision: wave 1, wave 2, and wave 3. It is only after a formal and often quite lengthy assessment period that children receive a 'Statement', and this only happens when the child is making very little or no progress, despite consistent interventions. In fact, very few children go on to receive a SEN. Most are supported by interventions put in place by the school, and some may access outside provision. The majority of children who go through the SEN process are not given additional resources to support their Statement. It is very rare for schools to admit a pupil who has a SEN in place before they start school to their reception or nursery class, even if they have been attending pre-school provision.

The various stages are the *Identification of Concerns* (the initial part of school action), followed by *School Action* and *School Action Plus*. This is followed by the formal SEN procedure. Table 12.1 illustrates the school's staged approach to responding to and recording the special educational needs of individual pupils in line with the SEN Code of Practice.

Table 12.1 The identification and assessment of pupils who may have special difficulties such as TS

Stage	Action
Identification of Concerns (the initial part of school action)	When a teacher is initially concerned about a pupil, he/she will discuss this with the parent/carer and complete an Identification/Concerns form, which highlights the pupil's specific difficulty, and also the strategies, which may help both at school and at home. The teacher then informs the Inc-co, and the pupil's name is added to the school's SEN list.
School Action	If concerns persist, the teacher will complete a School Action Individual Education Plan (IEP), detailing the specific targets and strategies to be used in lesson planning and any extra support which may be provided (e.g. teaching assistant support in class).

(continued)

Table 12.1 The identification and assessment of pupils who may have special difficulties such as TS *(continued)*

Stage	Action
	Both the parent's/carer's and pupil's views will be sought, and the teacher will discuss with the pupil (as appropriate) how he/she can be involved in his/her own targets and with the parent/carer about how they can contribute to helping their child at home. The IEP is reviewed regularly with the parent/carer and recorded on an IEP review form. Information from the IEP review is used to plan and set the new targets and strategies on the next IEP.
School Action Plus	If concerns persist the pupil will move on to School Action Plus. IEP and IEP review forms will be completed as above. Teacher, parent, pupil, and Inc-co liaise on provision as outlined in the Whole School Provision Map and specialist advice and/or support may be sought from outside agencies/specialists
Statement of Special Educational Needs (SEN)	If concerns about the pupil persist, the school may make a request for a Statutory Assessment to be considered by the LA. If the LA carry out a Statutory Assessment, the pupil may be given a SEN. Both IEP and IEP review forms are completed as above, in line with information contained within the SEN and a statutory formal review is held annually.
Statement of SEN process	Six parts as outlined in the text Three stages as outlined in the text
Successful SEN	Annual review Transition plan at annual review after 14th birthday
Unsuccessful SEN	Appeal tribunal must be within 2 months of LA's decision. Note in lieu of statement

Modified and adapted from the Special Education Needs assessment form at St John Evangelist Primary School, Islington.

A SEN is set out in six parts as follows.

1. Gives general information and details about the child.

2. Describes the child's needs and outlines any areas of difficulty following the assessment.

3. Describes all the special help and provision that could be given for the child's needs and also outlines monitoring progress.

4. Gives the type and name of the school the child should attend.

5. Describes any non-educational need the child has, which will be agreed by social services, health or other agencies, and the LA.

6. Describes how the child will get help to meet any non-educational needs (e.g. from health services, social services, or other agencies) and how they will be met.

Other difficulties can be recorded; for example, speech therapy can be recorded in parts 3 or 6, while transport must be recorded in part 6.

The SEN process is currently a three-stage process that incorporates and covers the six parts outlined above. A brief summary of the stages is as follows.

1. Discussions between teachers and parents or carers.

2. The school assesses the pupil's needs, which may involve the school's special needs co-ordinator (SENCO). During this the school discusses the pupil's Individual Education Plan (IEP) with the family, clarifying targets and how they can be achieved with special support. Many professionals may be included at this stage.

3. All the people (school, family, doctors, other professionals) involved in the SEN process meet face to face to discuss the child in what is called a Multi-Professional Assessment (MPA). If the SEN is not given to the child because the school feels that it is not appropriate, the parents have the right to contact the LA or appeal.

If parents/carers disagree with the Statement, they should first speak to their Named Officer or contact their Parent Partnership Service who can provide neutral advice and support. The right to appeal against the Special Educational Needs and Disability Authority (SENDIST) can be against parts 2, 3, and 4. The LA will be able to inform parents about local arrangements. Appeals to the tribunal must be made within 2 months of the LA's decision.

Other people involved in the SEN process may include, for example, an educational psychologist, an education social worker (ESW) (also known as an education welfare officer (EWO)). Individuals who may be involved in the education of a pupil with a SEN include a Named LA Officer, teaching assistants (TAs), and classroom or learning support assistants (LSAs). The TAs and LSAs provide support for an individual pupil or a group of pupils with SEN and/or disabilities. We believe that it is important for parents and pupils to know all these names and designations, as it is important to understand not only the process and delivery of education, but also that of the SEN and the plethora of new names that this involves. An independent parental supporter is available for any parent who wishes one. It is also useful to know that the government department responsible for the inspection of all schools in England is the Office for Standards in Education (OFSTED).

All pupils with a SEN have an Annual Review (to examine and ensure that all is going as planned), and a Transition Plan, in which steps and guidance are documented as to how best the child will progress from child to adolescent to adult are documented, is made at the first Annual Review after the pupil's 14th birthday. It is also important to know that there is a named person for each pupil with a SEN, who is independent and can give parents advice and help or act as their advocate. Finally, there is also a Code of Practice that gives LAs and schools guidance on their responsibilities to pupils with the SEN.

If the LA decides not to statement a child for special educational needs, they write a Note in Lieu of a Statement, which sets out the reasons for their decision not to make a Statement after the assessment.

It should be noted that parents/carers may experience difficulty at any stage, sometimes because the professionals have a different view of their child's educational needs, or, more commonly, because the process may be so protracted, with families perhaps having to challenge bureaucracy at every stage. Another frequent disappointment is what has become known as 'resource-led statementing', meaning that the Statement may be written only with regard to what funding is locally available, rather than to what the child actually needs. Therefore parents should read the Statement carefully to check that they agree with the details of the evaluation. We hope that the system will become easier for parents to use. It is a source of exasperation that they can well do without.

Finally, and importantly, there is the notion of pupil participation. The United Nations Convention on the Rights of the Child says that children who are capable of forming views have a right to receive information, to give an opinion, and to have that opinion taken into account in matters affecting them, and this is supported by the Code of Practice, which supports children being involved in decision-making processes about education.

Although the names of the processes and rules are probably different, we are aware that similar legislation is in place in other countries.

It is also worth noting that there are indeed educational assessments for children under the age of 2 years, but as TS usually begins between the ages of 5 and 7 years we will merely mention some of these: Early Years Action, Early Years Action Plus.

Administration of medication during school hours

As we have stated in a previous book (Carroll and Robertson 2000), it is often difficult to decide who should administer the medication to children during school hours. It is important to remember that parents are responsible for their children's treatment until they reach the age of 16 years, but there is no *legal* age limit below which a child cannot look after his or her medication. Thus, as we have said before, it is wisdom rather than law that dictates who should look after the child's medication. The best solution is for discussions to take place between the doctor and the parents, and then the parents or carers and school. The child should also be involved, if able. Many youngsters with TS know a lot about their disorder, and indeed their medication, and can probably administer their own medication. However, as they are at a school, it is probably wiser to examine the following possibilities as to who is best placed to 'manage' and administer the pupil's medication. These may include the following people:

- head teacher

- class or form teacher

- school nurse

- school matron

- school bursar

- school secretary

- parents/carers.

Types of schools and further educational institutes in the UK

It is important that the parents/carers of youngsters who have TS are aware of what types of schools are available. In the UK there are several categories of school that cater for youngsters with varying abilities. We will only list and explain some of these, as there are many, including for example academies, city colleges, and foundation schools, which are beyond the scope of this book.

A *mainstream school* is a 'regular' state 'comprehensive' school in which most people in the UK are educated and for which the parents pay no tuition fees. However, they may pay extra fees for some activities, such as outings. There are mainstream schools in every county borough and most pupils attend the school that is nearest to their home. These schools are under the jurisdiction of the LA. In the UK the mainstream religions such as the Anglican (Church of England) and Roman Catholic faiths run *faith schools*. The National

Curriculum is taught in these schools, but religious practices are also encouraged. In this context it is worth noting that religious education is a National Curriculum subject. A *grant maintained school* is a school that has opted out of LA control. The school has elected governors who run the school. There are also *Sixth Form Colleges* where students study specifically for A-level examinations.

There are also *independent schools* for which parents pay school fees. In the UK these include the public schools (which are, in fact, private) and others, such as Steiner schools.

A *special school* is a school that is especially for those pupils with Special Educational Needs. An *MLD school* is a school for pupils who have moderate learning difficulties. An *SLD school* is for pupils who have severe learning difficulties. An *EBD school* is a school for pupils who have emotional and behavioural difficulties.

A *pupil referral unit (PRU)* is an education unit for children who are not attending school (because of illness, exclusion, or other reasons). One of the aims of PRUs is to get the child back into school. They also have a wider brief, which is beyond the scope of this chapter.

Some parents opt for *home tuition*, and this may be the best way forward for a few individuals. It is important to ensure that home tuition is undertaken in collaboration with the authorities in order to obtain the best possible help for these few disadvantaged TS children. These may include those young people with severe loud vocal tics, loud coprolalia, violent motor tics, and constant touching of other people as a tic or compulsion, in addition to disruptive ADHD and non-obscene inappropriate behaviours (see Chapters 2 and 6). *Portage* is home-based educational support for pre-school children with SEN.

It is worth briefly outlining the mainstream educational structure. Youngsters usually progress through the education system as follows at the average ages indicated.

◆ Foundation (nursery school): age 3–4.

◆ Reception: age 4–5 (the 'bridge' between nursery and primary school).

◆ Primary school

  ◆ Key stage 1: age 5–7 (school years 1–2). Pupils in these years have teacher assessments in English and mathematics (often referred to as reading, writing, and arithmetic—the '3 Rs') as well as science during the year.

◆ Key stage 2: age 7–11 (school years 3–6). Pupils in these years have national Standard Assessment Tests (SATs) and teacher tests in English, mathematics, and science.

◆ Secondary school

◆ Key stage 3: age 11–14 (school years 7–9). At age 13–14 (year 8) the students have further SATs in English, mathematics, and science, and teacher assessments in other foundation subjects.

◆ Key stage 4: age 14–16 (school years 10 and 11). Most pupils take GCSEs or other national qualifications.

◆ Ages 17–18: examinations for further education are A-levels (the results of these are used on the UCAS forms for university entrance).

After leaving school, young people may attend institutes of *further education*:

◆ *Further Education Colleges*, from which the following *certificates* may be obtained:

◆ Higher National Certificate (HNC) and Higher National Diploma (HND), which are work-related (vocational) higher education qualifications. While university degrees tend to focus on gaining knowledge, HNCs and HNDs are designed to provide the skills to put that knowledge to effective use in a particular job.

◆ National Vocational Qualification (NVQ), which is a work-related competence-based qualification. NVQs reflect the skills and knowledge needed to do a job effectively, and show that a candidate is competent in the area of work that the NVQ represents.

◆ *Universities,* where one obtains a *degree* that can lead to a professional qualification in, for example, teaching, medicine, or law. Parents pay for this education or the student may be able to obtain financial aid from a bursary, loan, grant, or scholarship.

Can doctors help in the education of the student with TS?

First, we often *write formal letters* to schools and teachers suggesting that the child receives a SEN or, if not, we recommend measures that could help the child get better access to the curriculum. These measures may include one-to-one tuition at times, extra time for examinations or for completing assignments, using a calculator for mathematics, taking examinations in a separate room, and 'writing' the examinations on a computer. If the child also has ADHD and is disruptive, he may require 'time out' out of class to give his peers and the teachers a break. However, we point out that this 'time out' must in no way be punitive, as the symptoms are beyond the child's control. We also explain to the educators that we often prescribe medication for the children, which hopefully will reduce the disturbing symptoms. We have included an anonymised example school letter (Appendix 5) to give you an idea of how individual doctors can help.

Very occasionally members of our clinic *visit a school* to give a talk about TS—and often the school has more than one pupil with TS. These school visits are an ideal, but because of time restrictions are unusual.

Some international TSAs and Foundations and Tourettes Action (in the UK) are able to provide leaflets, videos and/or books on TS. This information can be obtained from your country's TSA.

What else can help?

The TS Associations and Foundations in Canada, and the USA and Tourettes Action in the UK have video films and educational books and leaflets about people with TS. Some schools and teachers find them useful for themselves as well as for the peers of the child with the syndrome. In this way other students can develop tolerance and understanding. In addition, these organizations have literature targeted at schools, and teachers are welcome to attend their meetings.

Many children with TS enjoy sport, and problems with tics and behaviour are often improved (i.e. less severe or frequent) during these activities. Ironically, the children are often better when they are concentrating hard on a task. Thus we encourage participation in sport if the child enjoys it, as this may be an area in which they may succeed and improve their self-esteem. As mentioned earlier, the famous American baseball player Jim Eisenreich has TS, and he has been a great inspiration to both children and adults with TS.

This reinforces our key message: encourage children with TS to concentrate on their strengths, and give them an extra large dose of praise and encouragement for those activities. Children (and adults) with TS may lack self-esteem and confidence. Therefore when they manage to suppress tics at an important time (e.g. during a concert), or when they do well at a particular task, this should be congratulated or acknowledged. This can increase their sense of self-worth, encourage them, and help them, and focuses not just on their condition, but on them, their achievements, and their individual contributions.

Useful websites for the SEN process and the National Curriculum

◆ Contact a Family http://www.cafamily.org.uk/educatio.html

◆ Dyslexia Parents Resource http://www.dyslexia-parent.com/statement.html

◆ http://www.direct.gov.uk/en/Parents/Schoolslearninganddevelopment/ Special Education

◆ http://www.direct.gov.uk/en/Parents/Schoolslearninganddevelopment/ ExamsTests

◆ http://www.direct.gov.uk/management/atoz/s/senidentificationandassessment

◆ http://www.direct.gov.uk/management/atoz/s/statementofsen/

◆ http://www.teachernet.gov.uk/wholeschol/sen/

◆ Qualifications and Curriculum Authority http://www.qca.org.uk/qca_ 5984.aspx

◆ The curriculum can be viewed at: www.curriculumonline.gov.uk

◆ The QCA provides a free online version of the curriculum at: www.nc. uk.net/

Education of the public about TS

Education of the public about TS is sadly lacking—very lacking. The majority of the media still highlight the swearing aspects of TS. We do not really like this, but we can understand why they do this as it is 'more interesting' as viewing or reading material and therefore it 'sells'. We acknowledge that if TV showed a programme about a boy who only blinked, shrugged his shoulders, and had a few other minor tics, sniffed and cleared his throat, was a good bright pupil and mixed well, went on successfully to secondary school and then university, and graduated with a good degree, it would (sadly) be boring to many. If he was also a good-looking fellow, played sport, and had a group of friends as well as a special girlfriend, had never sworn, taken drugs, got drunk in public, or got into fights, and had not been in contact with police, TV would be even less interested. We believe that he should be an inspiration and role model, but nowadays we are in a world of 'celebrity' and all the glitz and difficulties that surround many of these people—therefore anything 'ordinary' appears less newsworthy.

Currently in the UK we are very fortunate to have Tim Howard as the goal-keeper for Everton Football Club (the 'Toffees'). We remember that when he was signed by Manchester United, the press was full of negative publicity: 'F****** good goalie' and 'Man U goes for disabled goalie'. Since then he has received only good publicity, and has never been involved in a slur or scandal, which is the boast of few celebrities. There is more about Tim in Chapter 13.

We have also had Pete Bennett winning Big Brother in the UK—and he received more than 9 million votes and the programme was watched by many more viewers. He told the public that people with TS can be nice, warm, funny, and have fun—just like anyone else. He won Big Brother—no more need be said.

Employment

Employment and job satisfaction are some of the ambitions of almost every person on the planet. As we have stated before, people with TS can be doctors, teachers, or lawyers, or have any other job they choose provided that they are able and obtain the correct qualifications and training.

If an individual with TS has the correct qualifications, training, and experience, and believes that the only reason they not been appointed to a post is really because of their TS, they can resort to the UK Disability Discrimination Act 1995 (amended in 2005). It would be wise for the individual to discuss this with their doctor and Tourettes Action before launching out on what can be an expensive legal journey.

Sadly, however, there are some people with TS who are unable to work as their symptoms are severe, and it is important to know that there is financial help available in the UK. The NHS, general practioners, and the Citizens Advice Bureau (CAB) will know the details, but the financial awards and discretions are as follows:

◆ Disability Living Allowance

◆ Income Support

◆ HG2 and HG3 allowances

◆ Disabled Tax Credit

◆ Tax Credit Exemption Certificate

◆ Jobseeker's Allowance.

Any individual who is in receipt of any of the above can also claim travel expenses for NHS appointments. Each NHS hospital has their own rules about which and whom the patients should contact in the hospital. It is important for the patients to realize that although their doctors will be aware of these aids and transport refunds and payment, they are *not* the people to ask about the details. More information must be obtained from the CAB or the hospital authorities.

We decided to discuss these issues in detail because about 50 per cent of those with moderate TS have some employment issues. In addition, as we have shown previously, unemployed people with TS probably have a lower quality of life.

Empowerment

People with TS should know as much about their disorder as possible. Parents of children with TS should also know as much about it as possible. In our clinic, at the end of the initial consultation we give the patient and their family verbal and written feedback using our Feedback and Fact Sheet (Appendix 4) with all their symptoms described, all the scores they received on the clinician's and self-rating scales, and important information about TS and Tourettes Action (UK). We also give them a list of books, videos, and films about TS (see Appendix 2), and Tourettes Action (UK) flyer with all contact details. We believe that giving the patients and their parents information about TS makes them understand and able to reflect at home afterwards without having to resort to memory. We also feel that this is a beginning of the process of *empowerment*, so that they have some control over their worlds of TS.

We also tell them how to find medically acceptable information about TS on the Internet. The Internet can be browsed by anyone, but unfortunately not all information and sites give correct information. When doctors write an academic research paper it is submitted to an appropriate journal and then undergoes 'peer review', i.e. experts in the TS world look at the paper and make comments, and only after any recommended changes have been made can the paper be accepted for publication. Nearly all peer-reviewed papers on TS give solid information about TS, although some may be too scientific for most laypeople. However, most papers have short abstracts that are easy to understand.

We recommend that people familiarize themselves with these peer-reviewed publications as part of the empowerment and education about TS (and indeed any other medical problem). If you want to find out about these peer-reviewed papers, here is the method. Go to Google, type in Entrez Pubmed, and wait for the '16 million' hit. Then type in Tourette followed by any subject in which you are interested, e.g. 'Tourette cause', 'Tourette genetics', 'Tourette prognosis', and so forth. If you meet someone who says they know a lot and write a lot about TS, and you doubt it, you could always check by entering 'Tourette and their name (e.g. Bloggs)'!

It is important that all people with TS and their families become familiar with the Disability Discrimination Act 1995 (DDA) (amended in 2005) that gives disabled people rights in the areas of:

- education

- employment

- access to goods, facilities, and services

- buying or renting land or property, including making it easier for disabled persons to rent property and for tenants to make disability related adaptations.

The DDA also allows the government to set minimum standards so that disabled people can use public transport easily. The Department for Work and Pensions (DWP) website provides further information, including details of the alterations made by DDA 2005. The Disability Rights Commission (DRC) closed on 27 September 2007, but the website is still open and has plenty of information that may be of help.

Extra helpful information on TS

The UK governmental stance on TS

In the UK, members of the government recognized that TS occurs in 1 per cent of school children, as was exemplified by an Early Day Motion (EDM 1707), which was signed by as many as 99 members of the House of Commons on the 28 February 2006. This EDM correctly stated the symptoms of TS and noted that the signatories believed or acknowledged the following:

- It is probably inappropriate to serve patients with TS with anti-social behaviour orders (ASBOs)

- The national shortage of specialists for diagnosis and treatment

- It is concerned that requests for a SEN are frequently turned down by schools and by local education authorities

◆ Calls on the government to improve interdepartmental cooperation for patients with TS across health, education, employment, and social services

◆ Recommends a review of relevant research funding in the UK.

Empowerment also means that an individual with TS, or a parent who has a child with TS, or a doctor who has a patient with TS *can* do something to improve the quality of life of people with TS—with special relevance to health education and employment. We say 'If the cap fits wear it' and do something personally and nationally about people with TS. At times, the government responds to an EDM, but we were unable to find a government response to EDM 1707.

Driving and TS

It is quite natural and understandable for people with TS to want to drive a car. In fact, this is an essential form of transport for many people. TS itself is not a bar to driving in the majority of individuals, and indeed many people's tics improve when they drive (as tics improve when people play sport, dance, play music). However, the individual with TS in the UK should declare their diagnosis and any medication to the *Driver and Vehicle Licensing Agency (DVLA)* in Swansea (we often write supportive letters to the DVLA and know of no instances where an individual with TS has been refused a driving licence). It is also imperative that the driver with TS inform his/her *insurance company* about the diagnosis and medication, otherwise they might find themselves uninsured if they are involved an accident, even if they were not the cause of the accident.

It is also important to know that about 60 per cent of people with TS also have ADHD and it is often sustained into adulthood. There is research to show that teenage drivers with ADHD who are not medicated have more motor accidents and problems than other adolescents without ADHD. Again, it is important that the TS person, their doctor, and the authorities work together— to keep them and the roads safer places.

Expert witnesses and TS

A few individuals who have TS may need expert witnesses to help them in a legal sense. This may be because the diagnosis was missed (with serious and adverse consequences), treatment may have resulted in serious side effects, or the person with TS may, or may not, have committed a crime (which may be related or unrelated to their TS). Some experts on TS do not undertake what is known as 'medico-legal' work, but others do. It is important to have an expert witness who is really an expert in TS. Tourettes Action (UK) and most of the national TSAs or Foundations have lists of these experts, as do other associations. This information can also be obtained from the Internet, but an expert known to Tourettes Action (UK) and the various TS Associations and Foundations is probably the best option.

✖ Myths about education and employment and TS

◆ Most people with TS are in special educational schools.

◆ Most people with TS are unemployed.

◆ People with TS cannot drive.

13

Famous or successful people who have had Tourette syndrome

➲ Key points

Famous people who have definitely had TS and or tics include:

- William of Orange (1650–1702): King William III of England

- Peter the Great (1672–1725): the tsar who transformed Russia

- Napoleon Bonaparte (1769–1821): Emperor of France

- Dr Samuel Johnson (1709–1784): compiled the first English dictionary

- Tolstoy family: most famous member was Leo Tolstoy (1828–1910), Russian author

- Algernon Charles Swinburne (1837–1909): poet and critic

- André Malraux (1901–1976): French author and statesman

- Tim Howard (1979–): goalkeeper for US Olympic team, Manchester United, Everton

- Jim Eisenreich (1959–): American Major League Baseball player

There are many others—please see text

Introduction

It might be helpful to start by asking how we define 'famous' and 'successful'. Of course, fame is objective at some level, but there are simple guidelines such as being very rich, which is synonymous with being financially successful, or being a successful national or international player of any sport, which is synonymous with sports excellence. In addition, however, there are people who have done very well, but may not be well known outside their fields or countries. Nevertheless, there are many people with TS who have succeeded, and some have become very famous in their own countries, their own fields, or even internationally.

In addition it might be worth reiterating that many clinicians in the UK and USA in 2008 still erroneously believe that coprolalia is necessary for a diagnosis of TS to be made. We know that this is not true. Therefore when examining the lay and medical literature for people with tics, and especially TS, we are at a disadvantage as the diagnosis may not have been made correctly because of a general lack of knowledge about TS among both doctors and the public. Therefore we suggest that the number of famous people who have had TS is much greater than has previously been acknowledged.

It is also important to reiterate that many people have mild TS and do not know that they have it. Such individuals live quite unnoticed in their communities, pursuing their daily business in all walks of life. As in life in general, the majority of people with TS are not exceptional; they are 'ordinary' people getting on with 'ordinary' life. However, people who have severe TS may be severely disadvantaged, with few friends, and difficulties with employment, and as a result live with sadness and stigmatization because of what was erroneously called by many for years a 'very rare, bizarre and psychologically mediated curiosity'.

Dr Oliver Sacks has helped publicize TS for many years. In his books *The man who mistook his wife for a hat* and *An anthropologist on Mars*, he has given wide and sympathetic coverage to people with TS. Dr Sacks also described 'phantasmagoric Touretters' who seem almost super-human, with exceptional creativity, charisma, sense of humour, and productive energy.

However, there are many people who are well known, or indeed famous, who very probably, or absolutely certainly, do or did have TS. Many TS experts have met successful people, both as patients and on social occasions. These are not necessarily famous, but have done very well in their fields. We have identified medical doctors, TV personalities, and famous sportsmen who all do very well socially, but nevertheless have tics and make noises, and so, in the opinion of many experts, they actually have TS. Let us first see who might have had TS.

Historical figures with TS

It is perhaps best to begin with history, as several famous historical figures have almost certainly had TS or tics. William of Orange, who became King William III of England had asthma but was also described as having a 'chronic nervous cough' which was almost certainly a vocal or phonic tic. Others include Peter the Great, Napoleon Bonaparte, the Emperor of France, and the 'worthy Dr Samuel Johnson'. Another figure from Russia who had TS was Tolstoy's brother Dmitry (portrayed as Nicolai Levin in the novel *Anna Karenina*). Leo Tolstoy himself was a compulsive gambler, which many think may be a variant of obsessive–compulsive disorder (OCD). Therefore we suggest that the TS gene(s) could probably have been in Tolstoy's family. The poetry giant Algernon Charles Swinburne was thought to have epilepsy, but this was not true; he had tics and clear attention deficit–hyperactivity disorder (ADHD). More recently, André Malraux (French author, adventurer, states-man, novelist, and art historian) is also known to have had TS.

Contemporary people with TS

Many *well-known people* in current times have acknowledged that they have TS, and there has been speculation about others. These people include Pete Bennett or 'Perfect Pete' (winner of Big Brother in the UK in 2006), Kurt Cobain (American rock star), Mort Doran (a Canadian who is a surgeon as well as having a pilot's licence), Jim Eisenreich (retired Major League Baseball player, who has his own TS foundation in the USA), Noel Faulkner (come-dian and owner of art galleries and the Comedy Club in London), Peter Hollenbeck (professor of neuroscience at Purdue University in the USA), Tim Howard (the goalkeeper who has played for the USA, Manchester United, and currently Everton), James McConnell (British musician and author), Odd Nerdum (Norwegian artist), Pelle Sandstrack (Norwegian author, public speaker, and actor) and Julius Wechter (the marimba player of the 1960s American group, Herp Alpert's Tijuana Brass).

Some well-known successful *Canadians* with TS include Dan Aykroyd (actor, musician, screenwriter, and comedian), as well as Kellie Haines and Duncan McKinley whose stories we will look at in detail.

Other famous contemporary *Americans* who have TS include Mahmoud Abdul-Rau (retired professional National Basketball Association player, formerly named Chris Jackson), Eric Bernotas (Olympic athlete), Louis Centanni (comedian and author), Brad Cohen (author, motivational speaker, and teacher), Keith Collins (model and actor), Richard Paul Evans (author), Mike Johnston (minor league baseball player), Dash Mihok (actor), Luke Parkin (musician/composer), Calvin Peete (retired professional golfer), Tobias Picker (opera composer), Joshua James William Skaug (author), Ryan Slattery (actor), Jeremy 'Twitch' Stenberg (X-treme Motocross athlete), Steve Wallace (NASCAR driver), and Michael Wolff (jazz musician). Some neurologists also speculate that Thelonius Monk, the jazz musician, might have had TS.

We have space only to mention some of these people in detail and have chosen, in particular, those whom we have met and who have touched our lives, those who are extremely well known, those who have acknowledged TS, and those about whom we have been able to obtain sufficient information. We have also chosen those whose lives have taken very different paths since their tics began in early childhood. We have listed them in alphabetical order. The length of our resumé of their stories is not synonymous with their 'fame', and many have given us personal details that we hope will make their stories more interesting to readers interested in TS.

The stories of successful or famous people with TS

Peter the Great (1672–1725)

One of the earliest famous people with TS described in the scientific literature is Peter the Great, or Peter the First, who was Tsar (or Emperor) of Russia (Figure 13.1). He was born in Moscow in 1672 and became Tsar at the age of 10 years; therefore he reigned from 1682 to 1725. It has been said that he was a 'peculiar' individual and he has been compared with the Emperor Nero. He accomplished great things and was reported to be extremely intelligent, despite the fact that he did not receive a normal education and spent his youth in a small village with his mother. He was married at the age of 17 and had a conflictual relationship with his sister Sophia, who tried to have him killed.

Peter the Great implemented sweeping reforms and lifted Russia out of the Middle Ages to such a great extent, that by the time of his death Russia was considered to be a leading eastern European state. He is said to have 'westernized' Russia. He is acknowledged to have centralized government, modernized the army, created a navy, and formulated a very strong and aggressive foreign policy, as well as instigating many domestic reforms. He had a tough childhood, as during the Streltsy Rebellion and subsequent conflict, he witnessed the horrible murder of one of his uncles by a rioting mob. He won many wars, brought peace to many areas, and in 1722 created a new order of precedence named the Table of Ranks, which directed that precedence should thereafter be determined by merit and service to the Tsar,

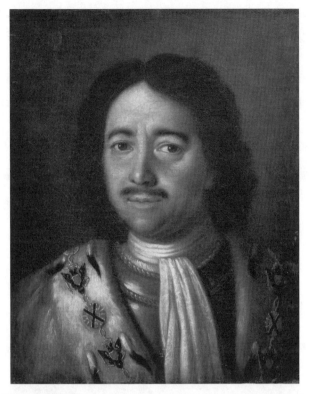

Figure 13.1 Tsar Peter I the Great (1672–1725), 1772 (oil on canvas), by Alexei Petrovich Antropov (1716–1795), Art Gallery of Taganrog, Russia. Reproduced with kind permission of The Bridgeman Art Library.

rather than being determined by birth as it had been previously. This continued until 1917 when the Russian monarchy was overthrown.

Peter the Great was acknowledged to have difficulties, such as problems with excessive alcohol consumption. However, he is also well documented as having had tics of the head and right arm as well as facial grimaces (making faces, wrinkling, screwing up his mouth, twitching his nose), all of which were apparently interpreted as a reaction to the various atrocities he had witnessed. It has also been said that he was very impulsive and, from time to time, aggressive. It has very recently been argued in a Swedish journal that he had TS. In 1679, at the age of 25, Peter the Great went incognito to Holland to learn the trade of 'shipbuilding' but was apparently recognized, as eye witnesses described him as being very tall (over 2 metres (6 feet 7 inches)) and with a broad figure and also described the tics of his head and right arm. He eventually died of kidney failure at the age of 53.

Dr Samuel Johnson (1709–1784)

One of the greatest scholars of the English language is someone of whom most people interested in the English language have heard—'Worthy Dr Samuel Johnson' (Figure 13.2). This literary giant, who compiled the first English dictionary, was also a famous poet and essayist. What the majority of people will not know is that there is no doubt at all that he had severe TS and severe OCD as well. This has been very convincingly argued and described in several papers in many medical journals by different authors.

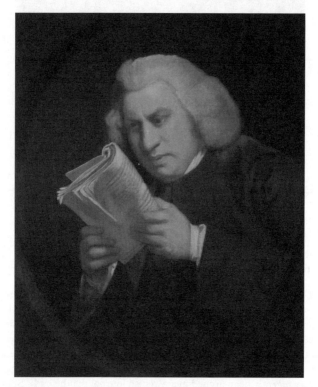

Figure 13.2 Dr. Samuel Johnson (1709–1784), 1775 (oil on canvas), by Sir Joshua Reynolds (1723–1792), private collection. Reproduced with kind permission of The Bridgeman Art Library.

Dr Johnson had many motor tics and movements, and also had curious vocal tics or noises such as whistling, chewing the cud, and the sound of a whale exhaling. He was a deeply religious man and did not have coprolalia, but did utter bits of the Lord's prayer out of place, which in those days must have been quite strange and possibly unacceptable. He also had echolalia (copying what other people say), self-injurious behaviour (he cut his nails deep until they bled), and severe OCD. In fact he had to walk in and out of a room until he felt that he had completed this action in the 'correct kind of way'. He also appears to have suffered from depression throughout his life.

Contemporary well-known, successful, or famous people with TS

Pete Bennett (1982–)

Pete Bennett or 'Perfect Pete' (Figure 13.3) exploded into British lives, homes, and hearts when he won the reality TV show, Big Brother, in 2006. When he began to participate in the programme in the house and 'diary room' many viewers expressed concern because of his TS. However, he won the public vote, and has become a real ambassador for TS, particularly in the UK. He nominated the UK TSA (this has now been renamed Tourettes Action) as his charity, came to their Annual Meeting in October 2006 and had his photograph taken, and also signed autographs for everyone who asked for the favour. He also held a question and answer session, and the audience was spellbound.

Pete was born in Peckham, South London, to Anne, a classical musician who also played rock music. She played with Siouxsie and the Banshees, a 'post punk and goth' band at the time, as well as many other groups—both busking and playing in theatres and on tours. Pete's Dad was Mark, an alternative punk musician, who often busked and who used to be able to 'talk in many voices at the same time'. Mark and Anne did not live together long term, and so Pete had several 'father figures'. Anne was always a loving mother, an independent lady, and she also had varied interests such as Egyptology and taking a course in music and visual art at the University of Brighton.

Pete was going to be named Sebastian, but after a torrid pregnancy, Anne, who had had a Roman Catholic Background, decided to name him after 'St Peter, the Rock'. As a child, from as early as the age of 5, Pete loved dressing up in numerous guises. He also loved Spiderman and had fun having his face painted as that of Spiderman.

Pete was diagnosed as having TS at the age of 10 years. He recalls the time he had to spend Christmas in hospital because of TS, and once even ended up in

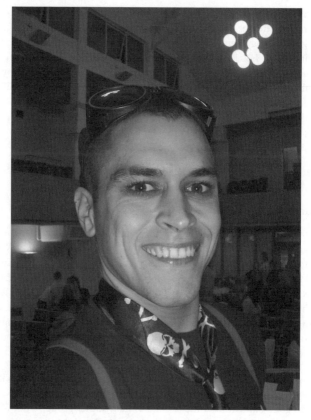

Figure 13.3 Pete Bennett. © Professor Mary Robertson.

a padded cell. At the age of 12 the diagnosis of TS was confirmed by one of the authors (MMR), who also diagnosed comorbid ADHD and OCD and took over his medical care for many years. After the diagnosis his mother, Anne, did as much as she could do for Tourettes Action. She persuaded a friend of hers who was the costumier in *Les Miserables* to create a Christmas tree costume for her, she wrote a song, made a CD, and went busking and selling her CD on the streets of London, collecting money for Tourettes Action, and her photograph was even published in *The Times* newspaper.

Pete also loved art, and Salvador Dali in particular. After obtaining his Art GCSE, he managed to get into Camberwell College of Art in South London, during which he went on a group trip to New York City. He had to obtain special permission from the American Embassy to be allowed on a plane and enter the USA because of his TS! When he was 17 years old, Pete painted an amazing painting for Jimmy Somerville, the rock singer, for his fortieth birthday. He studied at Brighton University for a year doing, as had his mother, music and visual arts, but then left as his writing really was not good enough and therefore he could not complete his essays adequately.

Because of Anne's musical career, Pete was brought up around people such as Jimmy Somerville, Marc Almond, and Lizzie-Anne. Therefore music was in his genes and in his environment, so to speak. It is not surprising that he was always interested in music and played the guitar with friends. He and a friend, Sarah, wrote songs for 'Turd Radio' at the age of 10–11 years. Anne married her long-term partner, Dave, when Pete was 11 years old, and Pete performed at the wedding reception as Freddie Mercury, wearing wonderfully wild bright crazy clothes. He also played the drums in a school steel band at Parkwood Hall. Pete then wrote his own music and eventually became the lead singer 'Daddy' in the Brighton band 'Daddy Fantastic'. After winning Big Brother, Pete helped Anne pay off her mortgage, bought his own home, wrote his auto-biography, lives with his long-term girl-friend, continues to play music, and has recently had a CD single *Cosmonaut* released. He has also formed a new band called 'Pete Bennett and the Love Dogs'. They regularly do gigs, and in 2007 toured the UK and Ireland and also played at Glastonbury. Pete has recently released a new music DVD, which is also available on the web. He has also given some of his book royalties to Tourettes Action, and on his 'Perfect Pete' website, there is the opportunity to donate to Tourettes Action UK.

Mort Doran (1940–)

Mort grew up in the 1940s and 1950s in Toronto, Canada. He was adopted aged 1 from a city orphanage. What he remembers most about his early child-hood is being obstinate and rebellious, with a rather prolonged 'terrible-twos' persona. He remembers being dragged kicking and screaming to the princi-pal's office in kindergarten at the age of 5. Much later in life, he was told by others that, on being introduced to adults, he kicked them in the shins. His tics began at about age 7 (although neither he nor his parents understood their significance)—first shaking his head up and down, then switching to side to side when told to stop, then eye-blinking, and then symmetrical shoulder shrugging. His parents were told that he was 'hyperactive', and would grow out of it. For the next thirty years or more a panoply of tics emerged, evolved, and resolved in a cyclical fashion, accompanied by disin-hibited emotional outbursts at the slightest provocation, a pattern of non-compliance and uncensored behaviours, made all the more trying and exhausting by a host of obsessive and compulsive time-consuming rituals that were stressful both for him and for everyone around him.

Despite these encumbrances, and in part because of them, he was determined and driven to do well at school. He succeeded, and then studied at medical school between 1958 and 1964 and graduated as a doctor. He spent five years in general medical practice, followed by a five-year surgical specialist training (residency), and began his career as a general surgeon in 1975, all the while doing his best to camouflage his tics, control his 'non-compliant behaviour', and keeping obsessive–compulsive rituals out of sight—in hallways, wash-rooms, and behind corners. Not until 1977, at the age of 37, did he ever hear the term 'Tourette's syndrome', despite having attended medical school for six years and completing a surgical residency. With hindsight, neither his pre-ceptors nor teachers appear to have been familiar with the disorder, for surely (he has asked them subsequently) they would have directed him away from a surgical career had they known—he was not *that* good at hiding his symptoms! His realization that he fitted the picture of TS came from a 15-minute discussion on a weekly radio science programme.

Over the past thirty or more years (he is now nearing 68) he has had a success-ful practice as a surgeon, and, other than being somewhat alarming to those who haven't met him, his tics, noises, and ritualistic behaviours have not been an impediment. He can easily control the tics while operating by incorporat-ing them into acceptable movements that do not appear out of place, i.e. read-justing his operating gown and gloves rather frequently and stepping back from the table from time to time to carry out some 'creative stretching'. Never has he feared that his erratic movements would cause him to 'zig' instead of 'zag'. In the same vein, while piloting his small Cessna aeroplane for forty years, never has he felt that any of his tics or rituals would intervene at an inopportune time to create any safety issue for his own or anyone else's aero-plane. It seems that he intuitively knows how and when to suppress these motor tics when required and 'save them up' for release when more appropriate.

Mort has now retired from active practice as a surgeon, and teaches the anatomy curriculum at the University of Calgary Faculty of Medicine as his 'retirement' project. His TS symptomatology has mellowed a bit (though not a lot) with time, and life is much easier now that he does not regularly have to struggle to 'prove himself'.

Would he have liked to have had a life without TS if that had been possible? Well, surely it would have been much less of a struggle, but fifty years of expe-rience in the medical field has shown him that there are innumerable diseases and afflictions far more consequential and debilitating than his moderate degree of TS symptomatology. In fact, the obsessive–compulsive nature of his personality has probably been beneficial in allowing him to have prevailed against the odds. So, too, can it be for all of those with TS.

One of us (MMR) has met Mort several times at TS meetings, and also in 2004 in Canada when he was given the 'Personality of the Year' award by the Canadian TS Foundation. Mort has, as one of his 'habits', a movement during which he touches people, especially their knees. We TS doctors have endless debates about whether or not certain movements are in fact tics or compulsions. Mary once asked him whether touching her knees was a tic (involuntary) or a compulsion (accompanied by a feeling of 'having' to do it). His reply was amazing: 'Sometimes it's a tic, at others a compulsion and I just have to do it, and at others I just like doing it!' That has taught Mary, and many to whom she lectures, that not everything an individual does must be a symptom of a disorder—sometimes it's just part of being a lovely human being.

Jim Eisenreich (1959–)

Jim Eisenreich is a retired American Major League Baseball player. He grew up in the small mid-western town of St Cloud, Minneapolis. His symptoms began when he was 6 years old, but he was only diagnosed at the age of 23, when he was already a professional baseball player, seventeen years after the onset of his tics. When his first tics (rapid eye-blinking) began he was given a diagnosis of 'hyperactivity'. Jim was interviewed about his personal account of TS in 1999 for a medical journal. He recalled that, from an early age, he knew that 'he was different from other children'.

Jim always enjoyed sport and participated in football, baseball, and hockey. He then became a professional baseball player and since his TS symptoms became publicly known, his achievement as a sportsman and person have made him a role model for other patients with TS. He started in the minor leagues in 1980, but in 1982 began playing for the Minnesota Twins as an outfielder. During this time a TS specialist recognized Jim's sniffing and grunting, but the Twins' doctors dismissed the suggestion as Jim did not have coprolalia. He was prescribed ineffective and probably incorrect medication, which led to unacceptable side effects. He struggled with his symptoms, played only from time to time for over two years, and had to eventually give up professional sport. Several years later another doctor suggested TS and prescribed haloperidol (a first-line medication at the time). Jim's symptoms reduced, he felt calmer, and he developed a little more self-control. He felt very relieved by his diagnosis. Jim also began to believe in himself again, resumed his professional Major League Baseball career in 1987, and has subsequently been regarded as a top defensive outfielder.

Over the years, Jim has won many accolades in his sport, playing for high-profile clubs including the Philadelphia Phillies, the Los Angeles Dodgers, the Florida Marlins, and the Kansas City Royals. Jim was involved with the American TS Association and began to help by talking at the TSA meetings and answering letters. In 1996 he founded the Jim Eisenreich Foundation for Children with TS. The mandate of the Foundation is to create awareness of the disorder and improve lives of children with TS. He stated that all his dreams have come true and he hopes that he can help the dreams of other people with TS come true.

Jim lives with his wife Connie and their children. One of us (MMR) has met him on several occasions, including in 1996 when he attended the national conference of the USA TS Association in California where he spoke and signed autographs.

Kellie Haines (1968–)

Kellie Haines is a professional ventriloquist, actress, and singer from Canada. She grew up in the small town of Wainfleet in Southern Ontario. Her two puppets Magrau (a bird) and Kamilla (a frog) also exhibited tics at an early age, leading experts to believe that they also had this colourful disorder. Today, Kellie and her puppets perform internationally for children and people of all ages in their educational show about TS entitled *Me, Myself and I*. Kellie does not exhibit tics on stage/set and has learned to focus her tourettic energy into her work and life. Her wit, compassion, and talent have inspired young people living with challenges to discover their own individual talents.

After many years of suffering with grimaces, loud noises, and body contortions, Kellie was hospitalized for six months at the age of 15 and it was only then that she was diagnosed with TS and put on medication. After graduating from high school, Kellie convinced herself that she did not have TS and ceased to take any medicine or treatment, leading to a second hospitalization at the age of 22. Since then she has come to terms with her disorder.

During training in music, dance, and theatre at the University of Guelph, Kellie was surprised to discover that her high energy could be utilized in her creative work. After graduating with an Honours BA in drama, she taught clowning and puppetry to young offenders, mentored children with TS, and continued her work as an actress in stage and film. She has puppeteered for a variety of television shows, provided vocals (theme song) for the popular children's cartoon Hamtaro, written and starred in two musicals at the H.R. MacMillan Space Centre Planetarium in Vancouver, and has a children's CD called *Songs From Space*.

Kellie is a recipient of the Richard Stein Memorial Award from the TS Foundation of Canada in recognition of the outstanding difference she has made in the quality of life of those living with TS. Kellie has been featured in countless radio and print pieces for her performance work, and she has performed with her puppets at many large events, including a mentor brunch at the Players Club in New York and at a TS Association America fundraiser where she met Oliver Sacks (whose work she has always admired). Although her symptoms can be painful, Kellie has learned that she is successful not despite but because of her challenges. She credits her TS as something that has helped her reach excellence in her work and life. Her parents and siblings have provided loving support throughout the ups and downs. Kellie met her husband, Greg Robinson, when they acted opposite one another in a play in university. They were married ten years later and live together with Magrau and Kamilla, and many other puppets, in Vancouver, Canada.

Peter Hollenbeck (1965–)

Peter Hollenbeck PhD wrote a moving, descriptive, and innovative account of himself in a medical journal in 1999. He described beautifully his 'endless and bewildering variety of irresistible urges, sensations, incessant internal drumbeats, background noise, challenging and enigmatic internal world' of TS.

Peter was born in 1965 in the USA. He vividly describes how, as he went off to his first day of school, in the second grade, his father watched him walking down the street, with his 'tics firing a 21-gun salute'. His father apparently sighed, imagining what his son would have to face in life, thinking 'Oh Lord, help him'. He and his father and family never discussed Peter's TS and tics, and their concerns were never voiced until thirty years later. Peter was brought up in a family full of love and companionship. His parents praised all his academic and sporting success, and thus he grew up feeling not only 'normal' but special, highly valued, and encouraged in his obvious academic prowess. He shares with the reader how, as siblings do, he was teased by his two older brothers—but the teasing was *never* about his tics.

Peter was fortunate, as in the early 1970s he was assessed and examined by a paediatric neurologist. However, this doctor did not give Peter a diagnosis or label, but instead saw him regularly, took an active interest in his academic life, and encouraged him to take up competitive running at the age of 13. The doctor told Peter that his tics were no more important in his life than athlete's foot. It seemed that the doctor genuinely believed this and therefore so did Peter and his family. The caring and patient doctor explained his ideas to the family and gave them a lot of personal time, calming and treating the whole family as well as Peter, the patient. It appears that this doctor was gifted. Years later, with hindsight and then as a neuroscientist, Peter believes that the doctor did what he did in Peter's best interests and he is grateful to him; there are many questions that Peter would like to ask the doctor if they were ever to meet.

Peter was diagnosed with TS ('his uninvited companion') as an adult by a leading neurologist. Peter surfed the Internet to learn about his medication, and his 'five little orange pills' reduced his TS symptomatology, which he found remarkable. Something that had been an integral part of him, such as 'ragged breathing with skipped breaths', was, with medication, reducing and disappearing. He talks about how, for most people with TS, 'their deeply rooted pain is not derived intrinsically from their tics, but from being tormented by others about having tics'!

Peter is a Harvard University graduate and is now a full professor of neuroscience at Purdue University in West Lafayette, Indiana. He has written books and at least 40 scientific articles, has been awarded grants to support research staff, and is also Co-Chair of the American TS Association's Scientific Advisory Board. We have met him several times, most recently at an international TS meeting in Lillehammer, Norway, in 2006, when he gave an inspirational talk from the TS person's point of view—he could not envisage life without TS.

Tim Howard (1979–)

Tim Howard (Figure 13.4) is famous in the UK, the USA, and internationally. He is without doubt *the* most famous living person with TS and is an

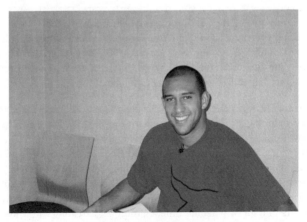

Figure 13.4 Tim Howard. © Professor Mary Robertson.

inspirational role model to all people. He played as a footballer (soccer player in the USA) for America in the 2000 Olympics in Sydney, was then goalkeeper for Manchester United (2003–2007), and is currently playing as goalkeeper for Everton (the Toffees) as number 24.

Tim was born in North Brunswick, New Jersey. He then attended the Montclair Kimberley Academy (MKA), a small private school in Montclair, New Jersey, finally graduating from North Brunswick Township High School. At school he participated in both basketball and football (soccer). He began his professional career soon after leaving school, beginning with the North Jersey Imperials of the United Soccer Leagues. He represented the USA in the 1999 FIFA World Youth Championship in Nigeria. What may be a little known fact to other than football cognoscenti is that, at one stage, he actually trained with AC Milan. He enjoys raising awareness of TS, and he invited more than 200 youngsters with TS to a match to watch him play. He has been known to say: 'Tourette's syndrome is not a problem. It is part of my life. It doesn't affect me one way or another on or off the field'. Tim has represented the USA at football 23 times (as of January 2008). He is married to Laura and they have two children.

He has won numerous awards in the USA including the Aquafina Goalkeeper of the Year (2001), Major League Soccer (MLS) Goalkeeper of the Year (2001), MLS Best XI (2001, 2002), and the MLS and New York Life Humanitarian of the Year (2001) for his work with children with TS. Other awards and accolades include being named English Premier League Goalkeeper of the Year in 2004. Tim is also a feature athlete and spokesperson for UNICEF and FIFA's 'Unite for Children, Unite for Peace' campaign. The American TS Association honoured Tim Howard at the 2004 TSA Champion of Children Award Dinner in Beverly Hills, California, but he could not be present as he was playing for 'Man U' so his mother, Esther, accepted the award on his behalf.

One of us (MMR) was fortunate enough to meet him in 2003 when he was given the Personality of the Year award by the USA TS Association. Again, he was far too busy saving goals for 'Man U' and could not travel to America to collect his award. Therefore, a group of us representing the UK TS Association (now renamed as Tourettes Action in the UK) travelled to Old Trafford Training Ground to give him his award. He was really wonderful, and was interviewed by a TV crew 'live' as he was given his award by a young representative of Tourettes Action. He also spoke to many of the other youngsters from Tourettes Action who had travelled to meet him, signed his autograph for everyone who asked for it, and allowed many of us to take his photograph.

Duncan McKinlay (1973–)

B. Duncan McKinlay PhD is a registered psychologist from Canada. He runs a clinic for youngsters with TS at the Child and Parent Resource Institute (CPRI) in London, Ontario—a dream job for a man with TS himself. He is a faculty member at two different universities, he is in demand internationally as a speaker, he has multiple publications behind him, he acts as a professional advisor for various TS organizations … and he drives a really cool car.

But it wasn't always that way. Once he was just Duncan—depressed, over-weight, alone, and undiagnosed. Duncan's 'secret' first became evident to him around the age of 7 when he developed a tic in his bladder muscles. Punished for repeatedly (and seemingly deceitfully) pleading that he needed to 'go to the washroom', Duncan began to internalize the message that what he was or felt was either bad or wrong, or both. Despite ever-increasing tics (such as humming, mouth-opening, and arm-jerking), Duncan worked hard to hide his symptoms from others and also from himself.

It wasn't until Duncan was 18, after years of counselling, family rifts, and a suicide attempt, that a newspaper article on TS by Ann Landers provided Duncan with an explanation and a direction. He soon went to McMaster University where he learnt everything he could about TS. He also began volunteering with a boy who had TS, and upon that family's insistence provided some community education and lectures on the topic.

Applying for graduate school was an uphill road, as university after university rejected the notion (and the applications) of a young man with TS who badly wanted to work clinically with children and spare them the kind of suffering he himself had endured. Eventually he was accepted by the University of Waterloo, but continued to experience resistance when requesting clinical training.

It was at this time, when all doors seemed closed, that Duncan's salvation came in the form of the TS Foundation of Canada (TSFC). Duncan was startled at the welcoming reception he received from this organization, and was stunned to receive their Richard Stein Award for making an outstanding difference in the quality of life for people with TS. With the TSFC as a touch-stone now providing much-needed strength and validation, Duncan persisted with renewed conviction in his quest to become a doctor.

It was not long before the presentation requests reached a point where a more formalized approach was necessary to keep up with the demand. Hence, Duncan devoted his 1998 Christmas holidays to banging away at the computer and his website 'Life's A Twitch!' was born. With the introduction of this website, requests reached a crescendo and soon Duncan was literally flying across the globe accommodating as many as 50 presentations a year. Then the media attention came. Then a documentary (also named, 'Life's A Twitch!') was filmed, coinciding with and actually capturing Duncan's PhD defence, marking his formal transition to Dr McKinlay. As the awards and offers began to roll in, the newly appointed 'Dr Dunc' found himself embraced as the professional that he feared for so many years he would never become. Perseverance isn't always a bad thing, it would seem! One of us (MMR) has met Duncan several times and always found him a serious professional (psychologist), great fun, and an inspiration.

Creating 'The Brake Shop' (the name Duncan gave his TS service) and acting as Clinic Lead is the culmination of fifteen years of dreams. Combining his training with personal intuitions and experiential knowledge has proved a very winning combination—within four years of opening its doors the clinic has been embraced by the community, recognized by the Ontario government, and identified as a Leading Practice in Canada. But, most importantly, every day now children can come to the Brake Shop, see Dr Dunc's example, and realize that they, too, can rise from the depths of despair to achieve their dreams.

Odd Nerdrum (1944–)

Odd Nerdrum is a Norwegian artist and figurative painter who has been speculated to have TS. He was born in Oslo and studied painting in both Oslo and Dusseldorf. He was apparently dissatisfied with the direction of modern art and so began to teach himself in a classical manner reminiscent of Rembrandt and in a direction opposite to that of his native Norway. He has devised his own approach to painting based on traditional methods, including mixing and grinding his own pigments, stretching his own canvas, and working from live models.

He lives in Norway but has made many trips to Iceland. His first single-person gallery exhibition was in New York City in 1983 at the Martina Hamilton Gallery. At one stage he was apparently somewhat controversial, and it was suggested that his work should be regarded as 'kitsch' rather than art. His work was featured in the well-known horror film *The Cell* (2000), which included a scene that was influenced by his painting *Dawn*, owned by David Bowie. His works are held in several well-known collections and art galleries including the Metropolitan Museum of Art (New York), the National Gallery of Oslo (Norway), the Gothenberg Art Museum (Sweden), the Kunsthal Rotterdam (The Netherlands), and the Amos Andersson Museum (Finland). Many books have been written about him.

Pelle Sandstrak (1965–)

Pelle Sandstrak grew up in Dönna, a remote fishing town in Norway. He dreamed of owning a car, and subsequently became obsessed with cars. When a car drove outside his school, he would gaze at the car, identify it, and then jump up and shout in the middle of the lesson 'Fucking asshole Saab!' Despite a strict upbringing he would find that inadvertently he would spit, swear, tell obscene jokes, and compulsively touch people. He had a phobia about the letter X, which he associated with fish-hooks, blood, and death.

Pelle has two sisters and an older brother; there are only three years between his sisters and Pelle. He told us that they all love each other and there are no family disorders or strange behaviours, with no known family history of OCD or TS. However, it has to be said, there have been quite a few 'characters' on his father's side. His mother always reminds him of that … and, as Pelle grows older, he can see his father's behaviour in himself.

When Pelle was 16, his father read an article in an English magazine about the odd behaviour of young people with TS and instantly he knew that Pelle had TS. His father organized an assessment with a psychiatrist in Trondheim, which was about 400 km away. After the interview the professor informed his parents that their son had an 'intractable personality disorder'. When Pelle's father disagreed, showing the doctor the magazine, the professor responded: 'Tourette's? We don't have that here'.

In the 1980s, Pelle moved to a flat in Oslo and his compulsions began to consume him. Something as simple, for most people, as going to the toilet would take Pelle absolutely hours and so he began urinating and defecating into plastic bags, which he hung from his walls, until all this became too much for him and he began sleeping rough. He discovered a car in a disused warehouse— a 1950s Chrysler of which he had dreamed—and for several months this became home.

Pelle tells of one day when his behaviour—strange ticcing, and crazy chatting—near his favourite hot-dog stand caught the attention of a producer from the local anarchist radio, who offered him a late-night slot. However, the producer had guessed wrongly! In the studio there was an envelope waiting for Pelle which read: 'A little something for you'. It contained speed from Poland and he found that, instead of giving him a rush, the amphetamine calmed him down. This was like magic. For the first time ever, Pelle realized what it was like to behave normally. The only problem was that Pelle was required to pay for the drugs, and the result was that he broke into a public office, stole 8000 kroner, and paid off his debts, but was then jailed.

In prison, with no speed to calm him and the jail routines making his obsessions worse, he was put in solitary confinement for refusing to walk through his cell door, as the guards deemed, 'properly'. In solitary confinement on his pocket radio, he listened to a talk show during which a professor described a boy he had seen who compulsively ticced and joked. Instantly Pelle knew it was himself and wrote a long letter, telling the man his story. A month later, the doctor came to find him. Pelle recalls that the professor from Stockholm was tall and slim, always chewing gum; he reminded Pelle of a sort of twin brother of John Cleese. Pelle says he will never forget him. After a few minutes he said, as if it was a question about cheese or ham: 'You have something called Tourette's. That's it'. The Professor took Pelle seriously and Pelle will never forget his words: 'I promise you Pelle. You will get a good life, you have a gift, you have a big heart and plenty of dopamine. Some people would kill to get that. One day you will get twice as much back from what you have been through. I promise you. Let's get to work.' When they met Pelle hadn't taken a shower for over a year. The professor saw his personality, not just the TS. Pelle had finally been diagnosed with TS, and for the next seven years was treated with cognitive behaviour therapy in Lund, southern Sweden.

Pelle is now a huge success. He tells his story publicly at conferences and also has a one-man theatre show. Always, he described how he had emerged from the wreck of an old car. A lovely thing then happened. Pelle was invited to open a conference in Chicago and amazingly the conference was sponsored by Chrysler, as a senior executive's son had TS. Instead of a fee he was given a gift, and now is the proud owner of a red Chrysler. He is now 42 and lives in Sweden with his long-term girlfriend Lina. In 2008 he published his book *Mr Tourette and I*. Outside his home stands his pride and joy—a red Chrysler.

Pelle now works as an author and public speaker, and freelances as an actor. He was recently in a Danish TV production, where he was intimate with a Danish actress, playing a young upper-class Danish woman living in a castle outside Copenhagen in 1834. Pelle played the gardener—they fell in love and out of love, but always conducted their secret body-tai-chi language in the castle's old park. Then her husband suddenly showed up and ... they killed Pelle's character. One of us (MMR) has met Pelle at two international conferences in Canada and Norway. He gave talks at both, and was a great success and inspiration to other 'sufferers'. At both meetings Mary and Pelle clearly remember Pelle touching ladies' earrings, including Mary's. Some of the women found it off-putting: Mary found it fun! Pelle has told Mary subsequently that he was a 'bit stressed out' that night, and so touching her earrings 'saved him a lot of problems'. He thanked her for her 'coolness and being a pro' (about her earrings being touched by TS folk).

❌ **Myth:** Mozart had TS

❗ **Fact:** Mozart did *not* have TS

Evidence for TS

◆ None.

Evidence against TS

◆ No motor tics

◆ No vocal tics

◆ No ADHD

◆ No OCD/obsessive–compulsive behaviours

◆ No positive family history

◆ No coprolalia

◆ His swearing was culturally sanctioned in his time.

Mozart deliberately wrote *swear words* in his numerous letters and music, and he also used foul language (scatology). No less than 17 per cent of Mozart's letters contained swear words (which were deliberate). In fact Canon 231 is called *Lech mich im Arse*—this was done on purpose and is very different from the rarely encountered 'involuntary' coprographia (writing foul words) in TS. *All Mozart's obscenities were done on purpose and indeed preserved for posterity.*

Appendix 1

An introductory card

One Tourette sufferer has a novel way of introducing himself in new situations such as on an aeroplane, on a bus, or in a restaurant.

Hi! My name is Paul

You may receive this card as a friend, employer or fellow student. As I have a visible and at times vivid neurological disorder, TOURETTE SYNDROME, I find this an easy, quick and necessary medium of introduction.

TS basically consists of involuntary movements and vocalizations—including obscenities. Symptoms can appear as outbursts.

All I ask is for you to see beyond Tourette to someone who in all other ways is normal and in many ways loves and excels at life.

PAUL M. SMITH – President, WA Tourette Syndrome Org (Inc.)

Appendix 2

Bibliography

St George's Healthcare **NHS**
NHS Trust

Tourette syndrome in the media and popular literature

We have provided a reasonably comprehensive, but not exhaustive, list of references to the media and popular literature for interested readers, under keyword headings. We have increased the list since the first edition. We hope that this will be useful for TS 'sufferers' and their families, as well as interested health professionals and students.

Films

The Tic Code (1998)

Dirty Filthy Love (2004)

Matchstick Men (2003)

Documentaries

John's Not Mad (1989) QED BBC2

Against my Nature (1990) Cutting Edge Channel 4

The Boy Can't Help It (2000)

Tourette de France (2006)

My Street: Adam's story (March 2008)

Televison

LA Law
Ally McBeal
St Elsewhere
Shameless

Books written by doctors and academics for the lay public

Bruun, R.D. and Bruun, B. (1994). *A mind of its own. Tourette's syndrome: a story and a guide.* Oxford University Press.

Carroll, A. and Robertson, M. (2000). *Tourette syndrome: a practical guide for teachers, parents and carers.* David Fulton, London.

Chowdhury, U. and Robertson, M. (2006). *Why do you do that? A book about Tourette syndrome for children and young people.* Jessica Kingsley, London.

Kushner, H.I. (1999). *A cursing brain? The histories of Tourette syndrome.* Harvard University Press, London.

Robertson, M. and Baron-Cohen, S. (1998). *Tourette syndrome: the facts.* Oxford University Press.

Sacks, O. (1986). *The man who mistook his wife for a hat.* Picador, London.

Sacks, O. (1996). *An anthropologist on Mars.* Picador, London.

Professional books (medical and educational)

Chase, T.N., Friedhoff, A.J., and Cohen, D.J. (ed) (1992). *Tourette syndrome: genetics, neurobiology, and treatment.* Raven Press, New York

Cohen, D.J., Bruun, R.D., and Leckman, J.F. (ed) (1988). *Tourette's syndrome and tic disorders.* John Wiley, New York.

Comings, D.E. (1990). *Tourette syndrome and human behavior.* Hope Press, Duarte, CA.

Kurlan, R. (ed) (1993). *Handbook of Tourette's syndrome and related tic and behavioral disorders.* Marcel Dekker, New York.

Robertson, M.M. and Eapen, V. (ed) (1995). *Movement and allied disorders in childhood.* John Wiley, Chichester.

Shapiro, A.K. *et al.* (1978). *Gilles de la Tourette syndrome.* Raven Press, New York.

Shapiro, A.K. *et al.* (1988). *Gilles de la Tourette syndrome* (2nd edn) Raven Press, New York.

Non-fiction and biography

Bennett, P. (2007). *Pete: my journey with Tourette's*. HarperCollins, London.

Byalick, M. (2002). *Quit it*. Delacorte Press, New York.

Fowler, R. (1995). *The unwanted companion: an insider's view of Tourette syndrome*. Silver Run Publications, Cashiers, NC.

Hughes, S. (1996). *What makes Ryan tick? A family's triumph over Tourette syndrome and attention deficit disorder*. Hope Press, Duarte, CA.

McConnel, J. (2007). *Life, interrupted: the true story of a life driven by Tourette's*. Headline Review, London.

Sedaris, D. (2006). *Naked*. Abacus, London.

Shimberg, E.F. (1995). *Living with Tourette syndrome*. Simon & Schuster, New York.

Wilensky, A. (2000). *Passing for normal*. Scribner, New York.

Fiction

Grafton, S. (1992). *H is for homicide*. Pan Books, London.

Hecht, D. (2003). *Skull session*. Pocket Books, New York.

Lethem, J. (2004). *Motherless Brooklyn*. Faber & Faber, London.

Walters, M. (2001). *The shape of snakes*. Pan Books, London.

Scientific bibliography

General reviews

Cavanna, A.E., Servo, S., Monaco, F., and Robertson, M.M. (2008). More than tics: the behavioral spectrum of Gilles de la Tourette syndrome. *Journal of Neuropsychiatry and Clinical Neurosciences*, in press.

Jankovic, J. (2001). Tourette's syndrome. *New England Journal of Medicine*, **345**, 1184–92.

Leckman, J.F. (2002). Tourette's syndrome. *Lancet*, **360**, 1577–86.

Robertson, M.M. (2000). Tourette syndrome, associated conditions and the complexities of treatment. *Brain*, **123**, 425–62.

Singer, H.S. (2005). Tourette's syndrome: from behaviour to biology. *Lancet Neurology*, **4**, 149–59.

Historical aspects

Itard, J.M.G. (1825). Memoire sur quelques fonctions involontaires des appareils de la locomotion de la préhension et de la voix. *Archives of General Medicine*, **8**, 385–407.

Gilles de la Tourette, G. (1885). Etude sur une affection nerveuse caracterisée par de l'incoordination motrice accompagnée d'echolalie et de coprolalie. *Archives of Neurology (Paris)*, **9**:19–42,158–200.

Lees, A.J. (1986). Georges Gilles de la Tourette: the man and his times. *Revue Neurologique (Paris)*, **142**, 808–16.

Meige, H. and Feindel, E. (1907). *Tics and their treatment* (trans S.A.K. Wilson). William Wood, New York.

Rickards, H., Hartley, N., and Robertson, M.M. (1997). Seignot's paper on the treatment of Tourette's syndrome with haloperidol. *History of Psychiatry*, **8**, 433–6.

Robertson, M.M. and Reinstein, D.Z. (1991). Convulsive tic disorder. Georges Gilles de la Tourette, Guinon and Grasset on the phenomenology and psychopathology of the Gilles de la Tourette syndrome. *Behavioural Neurology*, **4**, 29–56.

Clinical characteristics

Cavanna, A.E., Robertson, M.M., and Critchley, H.D. (2008). Catatonic signs in Gilles de la Tourette syndrome. *Cognitive and Behavioral Neurology*, **21**, 34–7.

Goldenberg, J.N., Brown, S.B., and Weiner, W.J. (1994). Coprolalia in younger patients with Gilles de la Tourette syndrome. *Movement Disorders*, **9**, 622–5.

Jankovic, J. (1997). Phenomenology and classification of tics. In: *Neurologic clinics* (ed J. Jankovic), pp. 267–75. WB Saunders, Philadelphia, PA.

Jankovic, J. and Stone, L. (1991). Dystonic tics in patients with Tourette's syndrome. *Movement Disorders*, **6**, 248–52.

Kurlan, R., Daragjati, C., Como, P., *et al.* (1996). Non-obscene complex socially inappropriate behavior in Tourette's syndrome. *Journal of Neuropsychiatry and Clinical Neurosciences*, **8**, 311–17.

Kwak, C., Dat Vuong, K., and Jankovic, J. (2003). Premonitory sensory phenomenon in Tourette's syndrome. *Movement Disorders*, **18**, 1530–3.

Mathews, C.A., Waller, J., Glidden, D., *et al.* (2004). Self injurious behaviour in Tourette syndrome: correlates with impulsivity and impulse control. *Journal of Neurology, Neurosurgery and Psychiatry*, **75**, 1149–55.

Robertson, M.M., Trimble, M.R., and Lees, A.J. (1989). Self-injurious behaviour and the Gilles de la Tourette syndrome: a clinical study and review of the literature. *Psychological Medicine*, **19**, 611–25.

Sachdev, P., Chee, K.Y., and Wilson, A. Tics status. *Australian and New Zealand Journal of Psychiatry*, **30**, 392–6.

Prevalence: how common are tics and TS?

Baron-Cohen, S., Mortimore, C., Moriarty, J., Izaguirre, J., and Robertson, M. (1999). The prevalence of Gilles de la Tourette's syndrome in children and adolescents with autism. *Journal of Child Psychology and Psychiatry*, **40**, 213–18.

Canitano, R. and Vivanti, G. (2007). Tics and Tourette syndrome in autism spectrum disorders. *Autism*, **11**, 19–28.

Eapen, V., Robertson, M.M., Zeitlin, H., and Kurlan, R. (1997). Gilles de la Tourette's syndrome in special education. *Journal of Neurology*, **244**, 378–82.

Eapen, V., Laker, M., Anfield, A., Dobbs, J., and Robertson, M.M. (2001). Prevalence of tics and Tourette syndrome in an inpatient adult psychiatry setting. *Journal of Psychiatry and Neuroscience*, **26**, 417–20.

Freeman, R.D., Fast, D.K., Burd, L., Kerbeshian, J., Robertson, M.M., and Sandor, P. (2000). An international perspective on Tourette syndrome: selected findings from 3500 individuals in 22 countries. *Developmental Medicine and Child Neurology*, **42**, 436–47.

Khalifa, N. and von Knorring, A.L. (2005). Tourette syndrome and other tic disorders in a total population of children: clinical assessment and background. *Acta Paediatrica*, **94**, 1608–14.

Kurlan, R., McDermott, M.P., Deeley, C., *et al.* (2001). Prevalence of tics in schoolchildren and association with placement in special education. *Neurology*, **57**, 1383–8.

Robertson, M.M. (2003). Diagnosing Tourette syndrome. Is it a common disorder? *Journal of Psychosomatic Research*, **55**, 3–6.

Robertson, M.M. (2008). The international prevalence, epidemiology and clinical phenomenology of Gilles de la Tourette syndrome. Part 1: The epidemiological and prevalence studies. *Journal of Psychosomatic Research*, in press.

Robertson, M.M. (2008). The prevalence of Tourette syndrome. Part 2: Tentative explanations for differing prevalence figures in GTS including the possible effects of psychopathology, aetiology, cultural differences, and differing phenotypes. *Journal of Psychosomatic Research*, in press.

TS around the world

Attah Johnson, F.Y. (1996). Gilles de la Tourette syndrome in Papua New Guinea. *Papua New Guinea Medical Journal*, **38**, 55–60.

Cardoso, F., Veado, C.C.M., and de Oliviera, J.T. (1996). A Brazilian cohort of patients with Tourette's syndrome. *Journal of Neurology, Neurosurgery and Psychiatry*, **60**, 209–12.

Eapen, V. and Robertson, M.M.(1995). Gilles de la Tourette syndrome in Malta: psychopathology in a multiply affected pedigree. *Arab Journal of Psychiatry*, **6**, 113–18.

Eapen, V. and Robertson, M.M. (2008). Clinical correlates of Tourette Syndrome across cultures: a comparative study between UAE and UK. *Primary Care Companion to the Journal of Clinical Psychiatry*, **10**, 103–7.

Eapen, V. and Srinath, S. (1992). Gilles de la Tourette syndrome in India. *Psychological Reports*, **70**, 1–2.

El-Assra, A. (1987). A case of Gilles de la Tourette's syndrome in Saudi Arabia. *British Journal of Psychiatry*, **151**, 397–8.

Micheli, F., Gatto, M., and Gershanik, O. (1995). Gilles de la Tourette syndrome: clinical features of 75 cases from Argentina. *Behavioural Neurology*, **8**, 75–80.

Min, S.K. and Lee, H. (1986). A clinical study of Gilles de la Tourette's syndrome in Korea. *British Journal of Psychiatry*, **149**, 644–7.

Robertson, M.M. and Trimble, M.R. (1991). Gilles de la Tourette syndrome in the Middle East: report of a cohort and a multiply affected large pedigree. *British Journal of Psychiatry*, **158**, 416–19.

Robertson, M.M., Verrill, M., Mercer, M., James, B., and Pauls, D.L. (1994). The Gilles de la Tourette syndrome in New Zealand: a postal survey. *British Journal of Psychiatry*, **164**, 263–6.

Assessment and diagnosis of TS and international criteria for TS

American Psychiatric Association (2000). *Diagnostic and statistical manual of mental disorders* (4th edn, text revision) (DSM-IV-TR). American Psychiatric Association, Washington, DC.

Gaffney, G.R., Sieg, K., and Hellings, J. (1994). The MOVES: a self-rating scale for Tourette's syndrome. *Journal of Child and Adolescent Psychopharmacology*, **4**, 269–80.

Goetz, C.G., Tanner, C.M., Wilson, R.S., and Shannon, K.M. (1987). A rating scale for Gilles de la Tourette's syndrome: description, reliability, and validity data. *Neurology*, **37**, 1542–4.

Goetz, C.G., Leurgans, S., and Chimura, T.A. (2001). Home alone: methods to maximize tic expression for objective videotape assessments in Gilles de la Tourette syndrome. *Movement Disorders*, **16**, 693–7.

Leckman, J.F., Riddle, M.A., Hardin, M.T., *et al.* (1989). The Yale Global Tic Severity Rating Scale: initial testing of a clinician-rated scale of tic severity. *Journal of the American Academy of Child and Adolescent Psychiatry*, **28**, 566–73.

Robertson, M.M. and Eapen, V. (1996). The National Hospital Interview Schedule for the assessment of Gilles de la Tourette syndrome. *International Journal of Methods in Psychiatric Research*, **6**, 203–26.

Robertson, M.M., Banerjee, S., Kurlan, R., *et al.* (1999). The Tourette Syndrome Diagnostic Confidence Index: development and clinical associations. *Neurology*, **53**, 2108–12.

Tourette Syndrome Classification Study Group (1993). Definitions and classification of tic disorders. *Archives of Neurology*, **50**, 1013–16.

Walkup, J.T., Rosenberg, L.A., Brown, J., and Singer, H.S. (1992). The validity of instruments measuring tic severity in Tourette's syndrome. *Journal of the American Academy of Child and Adolescent Psychiatry*, **31**, 472–7.

Wand, R., Shady, G., Broder, R., Furer, P., and Staley, D. (1992). Tourette syndrome: issues in diagnosis. *Neurosciences and Biobehavioural Reviews*, **16**, 449–551.

Woods, D.W., Piacentini, J., Himle, M.B., and Chang, S. (2005). Premonitory Urge for Tics Scale (PUTS): initial psychometric results and examination of the premonitory urge phenomenon in youths with tic disorders. *Journal of Developmental and Behavioural Pediatrics*, **26**, 397–403.

World Health Organization (1992). *International statistical classification of diseases and related health problems* (10th revision) (ICD-10). World Health Organization, Geneva.

Psychopathology, neuropsychology, and behavioural aspects

Bliss, J. (1980). Sensory experiences of Gilles de la Tourette syndrome. *Archives of General Psychiatry*, **37**, 1343–7.

Carter, A.S., O'Donnell, D.A., Schultz, R.T., Scahill, L., Leckman, J.F., and Pauls, D.L. (2000). Social and emotional adjustment in children affected with Gilles de la Tourette's syndrome: associations with ADHD and family functioning. *Journal of Child Psychology and Psychiatry*, **41**, 215–23.

Cavanna, A.E., Robertson, M.M., and Critchley, H.D. (2007). Schizotypal personality traits in Gilles de la Tourette syndrome. *Acta Neurologica Scandinavica*, **116**, 385–91.

Channon, S., Gunning, A., Frankl, J., and Robertson, M.M. Tourette's syndrome (TS): cognitive performance in adults with uncomplicated TS. *Neuropsychology*, **20**, 58–65.

Hounie, A.G., Rosario-Campos, M.C., Diniz, J.B., *et al.* (2006). Obsessive–compulsive disorder in Tourette syndrome. *Advances in Neurology*, **99**, 22–38.

Osmon, D.C. and Smerz, J.M. (2005). Neuropsychological evaluation in the diagnosis and treatment of Tourette's syndrome. *Behavior Modification*, **29**, 746–83.

Rickards, H. and Robertson, M.M. (2003). A controlled study of psychopathology and associated symptoms in Tourette syndrome. *World Journal of Biological Psychiatry*, **4**, 64–8.

Rizzo, R., Curatolo, P., Gulisano, M., Virzì, M., Arpino, C., and Robertson, M.M. (2007). Disentangling the effects of Tourette syndrome and attention deficit hyperactivity disorder on cognitive and behavioral phenotypes. *Brain and Development*, **29**, 413–20.

Robertson, M.M. (2003). The heterogeneous psychopathology of Tourette syndrome. In: *Mental and behavioral dysfunction in movement disorders* (ed M.A. Bedard, Y. Agid, S. Chouinard, S. Fahn, A.D. Korczyn, and P. Lesperance), pp. 443–66. Humana Press, Totowa, NJ.

Robertson, M.M. (2006). Attention deficit hyperactivity disorder, tics and Tourette's syndrome: the relationship and treatment implications. *European Child and Adolescent Psychiatry*, **15**, 1–11.

Robertson, M.M. (2006). Mood disorders and Gilles de la Tourette's syndrome: an update on prevalence, etiology, comorbidity, clinical associations, and implications. *Journal of Psychosomatic Research*, **61**, 349–58.

Robertson, M.M., Trimble, M.R., and Lees, A.J. (1988). The psychopathology of the Gilles de la Tourette syndrome: a phenomenological analysis. *British Journal of Psychiatry*, **152**, 383–90.

Robertson, M.M., Banerjee, S., Hiley, P.J., and Tannock, C. (1997). Personality disorders and psychopathology in Tourette's syndrome: a controlled study. *British Journal of Psychiatry*, **171**, 283–6.

Rosenberg, L.A., Harris, J.C., and Singer, H.S. (1984). Relationship of the child behavior checklist to an independent measure of psychopathology. *Psychological Report*, **54**, 427–30.

Sukhodolsky, D.G., Scahill, L., Zhang, H., *et al.* (2003). Disruptive behavior in children with Tourette's syndrome: association with ADHD comorbidity, tic severity, and functional impairment. *Journal of the American Academy of Child and Adolescent Psychiatry*, **42**, 98–105.

Termine, C., Balottin, U., Rossi, G., *et al.* (2006). Psychopathology in children and adolescents with Tourette's syndrome: a controlled study. *Brain and Development*, **28**, 69–75.

The long-term outcome (prognosis) of TS

Bloch, M.H., Leckman, J.F., Zhu, H., and Peterson, B.S. (2005). Caudate volumes in childhood predict symptom severity in adults with Tourette syndrome. *Neurology*, **65**,1253–8.

Carter, A.S., Pauls, D.L., Leckman, J.F., and Cohen, D.J. (1994). A prospective longitudinal study of Gilles de la Tourette syndrome. *Journal of the American Academy of Child and Adolescent Psychiatry*, **33**, 377–85.

Coffey, B.J., Biederman, J., Geller, D., *et al.* (2000). Distinguishing illness severity from tic severity in children and adolescents with Tourette's disorder. *Journal of the American Academy of Child and Adolescent Psychiatry*, **39**, 556–61.

Coffey, B.J., Biederman, J., Geller, D., *et al.* (2004). Reexamining Tic persistence and Tic-associated impairment in Tourette's Disorder: findings from a naturalistic follow-up study. *Journal of Nervous and Mental Disease*, **192**, 776–80.

Erenberg, G., Cruse, R.P., and Rothner, A.D. (1987). The natural history of Tourette syndrome: a follow-up study. *Annals of Neurology*, **22**, 383–5.

Leckman, J.F., Zhang, H., Vitale, A., *et al.* (1998). Course of tic severity in Tourette syndrome: the first two decades. *Pediatrics*, **102**, 14–19.

Pappert, E.J., Goetz, C.J., Louis, E.D., Blasucci, L., and Leurgans, S. (2003). Objective assessments of longitudinal outcome in Gilles de la Tourette's syndrome. *Neurology*, **61**, 936–40.

Peterson, B.S., Pine, D.S., Cohen, P., and Brook, J.S. (2001). Prospective, longitudinal study of tic, obsessive-compulsive, and attention-deficit/ hyperactivity disorders in an epidemiological sample. *Journal of the American Academy of Child and Adolescent Psychiatry*, **40**, 685–95.

The effects of TS on the patient and the family

Abwender, D.A., Como, P.G., Kurlan, R., *et al.* (1996). School problems in Tourette's syndrome. *Archives of Neurology*, **53**, 509–11.

Carter, A.S., O'Donnell, D.A., Schultz, R.T., Scahill, L., Leckman, J.F., and Pauls, D.L. (2000). Social and emotional adjustment in children affected with of Gilles de la Tourette's syndrome: associations with ADHD and family functioning. *Journal of Child Psychology and Psychiatry*, **41**, 215–23.

Cavanna, A.E., Schrag, A., Morley, D., *et al.* (2008). The Gilles de la Tourette Syndrome-Quality of Life Scale (GTS – QOL): development and validation. Neurology, in press.

Cooper, C., Robertson, M.M., and Livingston, G. (2003). Psychological morbidity and caregiver burden in parents of children with Gilles de la Tourette syndrome (TS) compared with parents of children with asthma. *Journal of the American Academy of Child and Adolescent Psychiatry*, **42**, 1370–5.

Elstner, K., Selai, C.E., Trimble, M.R., and Robertson, M.M. (2001). Quality of life (QOL) of patients with Gilles de la Tourette's syndrome. *Acta Psychiatrica Scandinavica*, **103**, 52–9.

Packer, L.E. (1997). Social and educational resources for patients with Tourette syndrome. *Neurologic Clinics*, **15**, 457–73.

Storch, E.A., Lack, C., Simons, L.E., Goodman, W.K., Murphy, T.K., and Geffken, G.R. (2007). A measure of functional impairment in youth with Tourette's syndrome and chronic tic disorder. *Journal of Pediatric Psychology*, **32**, 950–9.

Storch, E.A., Merlo, L.J., Lack, C., *et al.* (2007). Quality of life in youth with Tourette's syndrome and chronic tic disorder. *Journal of Clinical Child and Adolescent Psychology* 2007;36:217–227.

Possible types of TS

Alsobrook, J.P., 2nd, and Pauls, D.L. (2002). A factor analysis of tic symptoms in Gilles de la Tourette syndrome. *American Journal of Psychiatry*, **159**, 291–6.

Eapen, V., Fox-Hiley, P., Banerjee, S., and Robertson, M. (2004). Clinical features and associated psychopathology in a Tourette syndrome cohort. *Acta Neurologica Scandinavica*, **109**, 255–60.

Mathews, C.A., Jang, K.L., Herrera, L.D., *et al.* (2007). Tic symptom profiles in subjects with Tourette syndrome from two genetically isolated populations. *Biological Psychiatry*, **61**, 292–300.

Robertson, M.M., Althoff, R.R., Hafez, A., and Pauls, D.L. (2008). A principal components analysis of a large cohort of patients with Gilles de la Tourette syndrome. *British Journal of Psychiatry*, in press.

Robertson, M.M. and Cavanna, A.E. (2007). The Gilles de la Tourette syndrome: a principal component factor analytic study of a large pedigree. *Psychiatric Genetics*, **17**, 143–52.

Storch, E.A., Murphy, T.K., Geffken, G.R., *et al.* (2004). Further psychometric properties of the Tourette's Disorder Scale—Parent Rated Version (TODS-PR). *Child Psychiatry and Human Development*, **35**, 107–20.

Aetiology: suggested causes of TS

Abelson, J.F., Kwan, K.Y., O'Roak, B.J., et al. (2005). Sequence variants in SLITRK1 are associated with Tourette's syndrome. *Science*, **310**, 317–20.

Hyde, T.M., Aaronson, B.A., Randolph, C., Rickler, K.C., and Weinberger, D.R. (1992). Relationship of birth weight to the phenotypic expression of Gilles de la Tourette's syndrome in monozygotic twins. *Neurology*, **42**, 652–8.

Keen-Kim, D. and Freimer, N.B. (2006). Genetics and epidemiology of Tourette syndrome. *Journal of Child Neurology*, **21**, 665–71.

Leckman, J.F., Dolnansky, E.S., and Hardin, M.T. (1990). Perinatal factors in the expression of Tourette's syndrome: an exploratory study. *Journal of the American Academy of Child and Adolescent Psychiatry*, **29**, 220–6.

Leckman, J.F., Peterson, B.S., Anderson, G.M., Arnsten, A.F., Pauls, D.L., and Cohen, D.J. (1997). Pathogenesis of Tourette's syndrome. *Journal of Child Psychology and Psychiatry*, **38**, 119–42.

Lin, H., Katsovich, L., Ghebremichael, M., et al. (2007). Psychosocial stress predicts future symptom severities in children and adolescents with Tourette syndrome and/or obsessive–compulsive behavior. *Journal of Child Psychology and Psychiatry*, **48**, 157–66.

Martino, D., Defazio, G., Church, A.J., Dale, R.C., Giovannoni, G., and Robertson, M.M. (2007). Antineuronal antibody status and phenotype analysis in Tourette's syndrome. *Movement Disorders*, **22**, 1424–9.

Mell, L.K., Davis, R.L., and Owens, D. (2005). Association between strepto-coccal infection and obsessive–compulsive disorder, Tourette's syndrome, and tic disorder. *Pediatrics*, **116**, 56–60.

Rizzo, R., Gulisano, M., Pavone, P., Fogliani, F., and Robertson, M.M. (2006). Increased antistreptoccal antibody titres and anti-basal ganglia antibodies in Tourette's syndrome: a controlled study. *Journal of Child Neurology*, **21**, 747–53.

Tourette Syndrome Association International Consortium for Genetics (2007). Genome scan for Tourette's disorder in affected sib-pairs and multi-generational families. *American Journal of Human Genetics*, **80**, 265–72.

Neuroanatomy, neurobiology, and neurophysiology (how the brain works in TS)

Frey, K.A. and Albin, R.L. (2006). Neuroimaging of Tourette syndrome. *Journal of Child Neurology*, **21**, 672–7.

Hoekstra, P.J., Anderson, G.M., Limburg, P.C., Korf, J., Kallenberg, C.G., and Minderaa, R.B. (2004). Neurobiology and neuroimmunology of Tourette's syndrome: an update. *Cellular and Molecular Life Sciences*, **61**, 886–98.

Martino, D., Draganski, B., Cavanna, A.E., *et al.* (2008). Anti-basal ganglia antibodies and Tourette's symdrome: a voxel based morphometry and diffusion tensor imaging study in an adult population. *Journal of Neurology, Neurosurgery and Psychiatry*, in press.

Mink, J.W. (2006). Neurobiology of basal ganglia and Tourette syndrome: basal ganglia circuits and thalamocortical outputs. *Advances in Neurology*, **99**, 89–98.

Olson, S. (2004). Neurobiology: making sense of Tourette's. *Science*, **305**, 1390–2.

Peterson, B.S., Thomas, P., Kane, M.J., *et al.* (2003). Basal ganglia volumes in patients with Gilles de la Tourette syndrome. *Archives of General Psychiatry*, **60**, 415–24.

Serra-Mestres, J., Ring, H.A., Costa, D.C., *et al.* (2004). Dopamine transporter binding in Gilles de la Tourette syndrome. *Acta Psychiatrica Scandinavica*, **109**, 140–6.

Singer, H.S. and Minzer, K. (2003). Neurobiology of Tourette's syndrome: concepts of neuroanatomic localization and neurochemical abnormalities. *Brain and Development*, **25** (Suppl 1), S70–84.

Stern, E., Silbersweig, D.A., Chee, K.-Y., *et al.* (2000). A functional neuroanatomy of tics in Tourette syndrome. *Archives of General Psychiatry*, **57**, 741–8.

Voelker, R. (2004). Scientists use neuroimaging, genetic studies to probe biology of Tourette syndrome. *Journal of the American Medical Association*, **292**, 909–11.

Treatment

Gilbert, D. (2006). Treatment of children and adolescents with tics and Tourette syndrome. *Journal of Child Neurology*, **21**, 690–700.

Himle, M.B., Woods, D.W., Piacentini, J.C., and Walkup, J.T. (2006). Brief review of habit reversal training for Tourette syndrome. *Journal of Child Neurology*, **21**, 719–25.

Neimat, J.S., Patil, P.G., and Lozano, A.M. (2006). Novel surgical therapies for Tourette syndrome. *Journal of Child Neurology*, **21**, 715–18.

Orth, M., Kirby, R., Richardson, M.P., *et al.* (2005). Subthreshold rTMS over pre-motor cortex has no effect on tics in patients with Gilles de la Tourette syndrome. *Clinical Neurophysiology*, **116**, 764–8.

Peterson, B.S. and Cohen, D.J. (1998). The treatment of Tourette's syndrome: multimodal, developmental intervention. *Journal of Clinical Psychiatry*, **59** (Suppl 1), S62–72.

Scahill, L., Erenberg, G., Berlin, C.M., Jr, *et al.* (2006). Tourette syndrome Association Medical Advisory Board: Practice Committee. Contemporary assessment and pharmacotherapy of Tourette syndrome. *NeuroRx*, **3**, 192–206.

Scott, B.L., Jankovic, J., and Donovan, D.T. (1996). Botulinum toxin injection into vocal cord in the treatment of malignant coprolalia associated with Tourette's syndrome. *Movement Disorders*, **11**, 431–3.

Servello, D., Porta, M., Sassi, M., Brambilla, A., and Robertson, M.M. (2008). Deep brain stimulation in 18 patients with severe Gilles de la Tourette syndrome refractory to treatment: the surgery and stimulation. *Journal of Neurology, Neurosurgery and Psychiatry*, **79**, 136–42.

Visser-Vandewalle, V. (2007). DBS in Tourette syndrome: rationale, current status and future prospects. *Acta Neurochirurgica Supplementum*, **97**, 215–22.

Visser-Vandewalle, V., van der Linden, C.H.R, Groenewegen, H.J., and Caemaert, J. (1999). Stereotactic treatment of Gilles de la Tourette syndrome by high frequency stimulation of thalamus. *Lancet*, **353**, 724.

Well known, famous, or successful people with TS

Fuerst, M.L. (1999). An interview with Jim Eisenreich. *CNS Spectrums*, **4**,18.

Hollenbeck, P (1999). How life imitates Tourette syndrome: reflections of an afflicted neuroscientist. *CNS Spectrums*, **4**, 22–3.

Hurst, M.J. and Hurst, D.L. (1994). Tolstoy's description of Tourette syndrome in *Anna Karenina. Journal of Child Neurology*, **94**, 366–7.

Lagerkvist, B. (2005). Peter the Great and Tourette syndrome: impulsive, violent sovereign who drank a lot of alcohol to control his tics. *Lakartidningen*, **102**, 1440–3.

McHenry, L.C., Jr (1967). Samuel Johnson's tics and gesticulations. *Journal of the History of Medicine*, **22**, 152–68.

Murray, T.J. (1979). Dr Samuel Johnson's movement disorder. *British Medical Journal*, **1**, 1610–14.

Pearce, J.M. (1994). Doctor Samuel Johnson, 'the great convulsionary': a victim of Gilles de la Tourette's syndrome. *Journal of the Royal Society of Medicine*, **87**, 396–9.

Rickards, H. (1995). Tics and fits: the current status of Gilles de la Tourette syndrome and its relationship with epilepsy. *Seizure*, **4**, 259–66.

Web resources

http://en.wikipedia.org/wiki/Tourette

http://www.emedicine.com/neuro/topic664.htm

http://www.tourette-confusion.blogspot.com

http://www.timeout.com/London/comedy/features/1601.html

Appendix 3

Tourette syndrome international contacts and associations

Argentina

Guillermo Tyberg

Williams 1.800

Barrio Los Ceibos

Rincon De Milberg

B1624EJB Tigre

Prov. de Buenos Aires, Argentina

Tel/Fax: +54-911-4749-8660

Mobile: +54-911-5469-5133

Email: gtyberg@fibertel.com.ar

Australia

Tourette Syndrome Association of Australia Inc.

PO Box 1173

Maroubra, NSW 2035, Australia

President: Russell Oxford

Vice-President: Elizabeth Burns

Tel: +61-2-9382-3726

Fax: +61-2-9382-3764

Email: info@tourette.org.au

Tourette Syndrome Association of Victoria Inc.

The Nerve Centre

54 Railway Road

Blackburn, Vic 3130, Australia

Tel: + 03-9845-2700

Fax: + 03-9845-2777

Email: tourettes@mssociety.com.au

Website: www.tsavic.org.au

Austria

Univ. Prof. Dr. Mara Stamenkovic

Department for Biological Psychiatry

Medical University Vienna

Währinger Gürtel 18-20

A-1090 Vienna, Austria

Tel.: +43-1-40400-3501

Fax: +43-1-40400-3560

Mobile: +43-676-517-9057

Email: mara.stamenkovic@meduniwien.ac.at

Belgium

Gilles de la Tourette

President: Vera Casier-Cassimon (Flemish)

vzw Vlaamse Vereniging Gilles de la Tourette

J. Nauwelaertstraat 7

2210 Wijnegem, Belgium

Tel: +32-3-354-3669

Fax: +32-3-353-6791

Email: info@tourette.be

Website: www.tourette.be

Brazil

Euripedes C. Miguel, MD, PhD
PROTOC do IPQ-HCFMUSP
Rua Ovidio Pires de Campos, s/n° - sala 4025
05403-010 Sao Paulo, SP, Brazil
Tel/Fax: +55-11-853-3531
Email: ecmiguel@usp.br

Bulgaria

Dr Dimiter Terziev
Assistant Professor
University Hospital Aleksandrovska
Child Psychiatry Clinic
1 Georgi Sofiiski Str.
1431-Sofia, Bulgaria
Tel: +359-9230375 or +359-9230681
Email: dislter@yahoo.co.uk

Canada

TS Foundation of Canada
194 Jarvis St., #206
Toronto, ON
Canada M5B 2B7
Tel: +1-416-861-8398
Fax: +1-416-861-2472
Email: tsfc@tourette.ca
Website: www.tourette.ca

Denmark

Dansk Tourette Forening (Danish Tourette Association)
President: Kirsten Kristensen
Søllerødvej 76
2840 Holte, Denmark
Email: kk@tourette.dk

Dr Anne Korsgaard
Specialist in Neurology
Skt. Anne Plads 2
5000 Odense C, Denmark
Email: agk@dadlnet.dk

Estonia

Pille Taba MD PhD
Associate Professor of Neurology
Department of Neurology and Neurosurgery
University of Tartu
Puusepa 2
Tartu 51014, Estonia
Tel: +372-7-318-512
Fax: +372-7-318-509
Email: Pille.Taba@kliinikum.ee

France

Association Française Syndrome Gilles de la Tourette (AFSGT)
President: Marie-Christine Biron
9, rue Louis Haussman
Versaille 78000, France
Tel. +33-1-39-50-1000 or +33-4-7687-4970
Fax: +33-1-4115-0845
Email: afsgtjfm@aol.com
Website: http://afsgt-tourette-france.org/

Germany

Tourette Gesellschaft Deutschland
Professor Dr A. Rothenberger
Universität Gottingen Kinder- und Jugendpsychiatrie
von Siebold Str. 5
37075 Göttingen, Germany

Email: arothen@gwdg.de

Website: www.tourette-gesellschaft.de

Hungary

Zsanett Tarnok

Vadaskert Child and Adolescent Psychiatry

Huvosvolgyi ut 116

H-1021 Budapest, Hungary

Tel: +36-1-392-1400 or +36-70-370-8429

Fax: 36-1-392-1411

Email: tarnok@vadasnet.hu

Website: www.vadaskertalapitvany.hu

Iceland

Icelandic Tourette Association

Director: Sigrún Gunnarsdóttir

Hátun 10b

IS-105 Reykjavík, Iceland

Tel: +354-840-2210

Email: tourette@tourette.is

Website: www.tourette.is

India

Dr Bhaskara Pillai Shelley

Head, Department of Neurology

Father Muller Medical College

Kankanady

Mangalore 575 002

Karnataka, India

Tel: 0091-824-2238331

Email: bpshelley@yahoo.com

Ireland

Tourette Syndrome Association of Ireland

Carmichael Centre

North Brunswick Street

Dublin 7, Ireland

Tel: 01-8725550

Email: info@tsai.ie

Website: www.tsai.ie

Italy

Associazione Italiana Sindrome di Tourette e Disturbi Correlati (AIST) Onlus

Policlinico San Marco

Corso Europa 7

Bergamo-Zingonia, Italy

IRCCS Galeazzi

Via R. Galeazzi 4

Milan, Italy

Tel: +39-3588-6298

Fax:+39-3588-5789

Email: aistonlus@virgilio.it

Website: www.tourette.it

Professor Mauro Porta

Movement Disorders Clinic and Tourette Center

IRCCS Galeazzi

Via R. Galeazzi 4

Milan, Italy

Tel: +39-2662-14903 Fax:+39-2662-14916

Consultations: +39-2662-141

Email: portamilano@libero.it

Professor Renata Rizzo MD PhD
Professor of Paediatrics
University of Catania
Catania, Italy
Tel: +39-95-256-464
Email: rerizzo@unict.it

Japan

Segawa Neurological Clinic for Children
2–8 Surugadai Kanda Chiyodaku
Tokyo 101-0062, Japan
Tel: +81-3-3294-0371
Fax: +81-3-3294-0290
Potential patients contact:
Segawa Neurological Clinic for Children
Director: Masaya Segawa MD

Netherlands

Dr Danielle Cath
Email: daniellc@ggzba.nl; cath@xs4all.nl

New Zealand

May Cross
Email: mayc@maxnet.co.nz

Norway

Norsk Tourette Forening
Postboks 4568, Nydalen
0404 Oslo, Norway
Tel: +47-2279-9414
Fax:+47-2279-9449
Email: post@touretteforeningen.no
Website: www.touretteforeningen.no

Philippines

Philippine Tourette Syndrome Association (PTSA)
Maria Rowena B. Victorino RN, BSN
Tel: +63-906-4960921
Email: ticawaywithme@gmail.com

Marlon Barnuevo
B-20, l-27 Reyes Ave
Greenfields-I Novaliches
Quezon City 1123, Philippines
Tel: +63-2-937-0911
Email: barnuevo@yahoo.com
Website: www.rxpinoy.com/ptsa/

South Africa

Professor Dan Stein
Chairman, Department of Psychiatry and Mental Health
University of Cape Town
South Africa
Email: dan.stein@curie.uct.ac.za

Tourette's Disorder Information and Support
Roberta Williams (Somerset West)
Tel: +27-82-924-4909
Email: chukiwilliams@absamail.co.za

Spain

Esther Cubo MD
Neurology Department
Hospital General Yague
Burgos, Spain
Tel: +34-947281922
Fax: +34-947281965
Email: esthercub@wanadoo.es

Sweden

Child Neuropsychiatry
The Queen Silvia Children's Hospital
Göteborg, Sweden
Email: bjorn.kadesjo@vgregion.se

Attention
Förmansvägen 2
117 43 Stockholm, Sweden
Tel: +46-8-709-22-60
Fax: +46-8-709-22-69
Email: kansliet@attention-riks.se
Website/Hemsida: www.attention-riks.se

Switzerland

Tourette Gesellschaft Schweiz (Deutsch)
Tourette-Romandie (Francais)
Website: http://www.tourette.ch

Taiwan

Dr Huei-Shyong Wang MD
Chang Gung Children's Hospital
5 Fusing St.
Kueisun, Taoyuan 333
Taiwan
Mobile: +886-968110264
web site: www.ttfa.org.tw

Turkey

Yanki Yazgan MD
Professor of Child, Adolescent and Adult Psychiatry
Marmara University Faculty of Medicine
Istanbul, Turkey
Email: yanki@yankiyazgan.com; yanki.yazgan@yale.edu

United Arab Emirates

Professor Valsamma Eapen PhD, FRCPsych, FRANZCP

Previously Professor and Consultant Psychiatrist, Faculty of Medicine and Health Sciences, University of the UAE

Currently Chair of Infant, Child and Adolescent Psychiatry, UNSW, Sydney, Australia

Tel: +61-488785133

Email: valsa_eapen@hotmail.com

United Kingdom

Tourettes Action

Executive Director: Judith Kidd

Southbank House

Black Prince Road

London, SE1 7SJ, UK

Tel: +44-20-7793-2356

Helpline: +44-845-458-1252

Email: help@tourettes-action.org.uk

Website: http://www.tourettes-action.org.uk

Tourette Scotland

Algo Business Centre

Glenearn Road

Perth PH2 0NJ, Scotland

Tel/Fax: +44-1738-450411

Email: info@tourettescotland.org

Website: www.tourettescotland.org

United States of America

Tourette Syndrome Association Inc

42–40 Bell Boulevard

Bayside, NY 11361, USA

Tel: +1-718-224-2999

Fax: +1-718-279-9596

Appendix 4

Feedback Form and Fact Sheet

St George's Healthcare **NHS**
NHS Trust

Gilles de la tourette syndrome (Tourette syndrome: GTS: TS)

Patient's name =

Criteria   American Psychiatric Association (DSM-IV-TR) – 2000)

World Health Organisation (ICD – 10 – 1992)

Essential Features

Multiple motor tics: n = (ever): n = (at interview): n =(in last week)

One or more vocal (phonic) tics: n = (ever): n = (at interview): n = (in last week)

Coprolalia (swearing tic)	yes/no
Copropraxia (rude gesture tic)	yes/no
Echolalia (copying other's noises, words as a tic)	yes/no
Echopraxia (copying other's tics, expressions as a tic)	yes/no
Palilalia (repeating oneself as a tic)	yes/no
Attention deficit–hyperactivity disorder (ADHD)	yes/no

Obsessive–compulsive behaviours (OCB)	yes/no
Obsessive–compulsive disorder (OCD)	yes/no
Self-injurious behaviours (SIB)	yes/no
Oppositional defiant disorder (ODD)	yes/no
Conduct disorder (CD)	yes/no
Autistic spectrum disorder (ASD) e.g. Asperger's, autism	yes/no
Depressive illness	yes/no
Cause – genetic	yes/no
– peri-natal complications	yes/no
– PANDAS hypothesis (streptococcal infections)	yes/no
Yale Global Tic Severity Rating Scale	……%
Diagnostic Confidence Index	…… %
MOVES	……/60
Summary	mild/moderate/severe

Management

1. Explanation and reassurance

TS has no relationship to life-span

TS has no relationship to psychosis (e.g. schizophrenia)

TS often improves with age (by 18 years)

TS is common—1% of population

TS is very common in people with ASD (6–11%) and special educational needs

2. Education and employment

Normal

Extra help in examinations

Statement of Special Educational Needs

Letter—with written consent

3. Medication

Neuroleptics

Clonidine

SSRIs

Stimulants

Others

4. Behavioural treatments

Habit reversal training

Cognitive-behaviour therapy

Psychotherapy

Counselling

5. Other treatments

6. Tourettes Action

Southbank House, Black Prince Road, London, SE1 7SJ

Tel:: +44 20 7793 2356

Telephone Helpline: +44 845 458 1252

Email: help@tourettes-action.org.uk

7. Information

(a) ENTREZ PUBMED (Peer review papers on TS)

Google > entrez pubmed > 16 million citations > Tourette + subject

(b) Papers and information on TS (separate pages)

TS Clinic doctors at St George's Hospital

Prof Mary M. Robertson .... Signature .... Date ....

Dr Helen Simmons .... Signature .... Date ....

Dr Jeremy S. Stern .... Signature .... Date ....

Appendix 5

School letter

Mr William Watson

Head Teacher

St Peregrine School

London SW20 7AQ

Dear Mr Watson

Re: Johnny Logan, 39 5th Street, Lower Houghton, London SW3 39FR

Johnny has attended our clinic for the Gilles de la Tourette syndrome and related disorders, and his parents have asked me to write to you with what I hope will be some information useful in managing this problem in the classroom.

I diagnosed the primary illness as the Gilles de la Tourette syndrome. In addition Johnny also has attention deficit–hyperactivity disorder (ADHD) and obsessive–compulsive disorder (OCD) (using the standard diagnostic definitions).

Tourette syndrome is a disorder in which individuals have multiple motor tics and one or more vocal tics (noises) which last longer than a year, and it begins in childhood. The tics characteristically change over time involving various parts of the body. Only a minority of people with Tourette syndrome suffer from involuntary swearing and Johnny does have this feature. It is very important to note that this is wholly different from excessive swearing in a social context (e.g. only when arguing) or unruly and nasty behaviour. People with Tourette syndrome who have this symptom find it very unpleasant and embarrassing, and often try to cover up the fact (e.g. by coughing).

It is important to note that youngsters with Tourette syndrome cannot help their tics. However, the movements and noises may be situational or voluntarily suppressible for short periods. It is a well-recognized medical disorder, there is treatment which is effective in some cases, and many strategies for helping youngsters with this problem.

Tourette syndrome is often associated with attention deficit–hyperactivity disorder and obsessive–compulsive disorder. In Johnny's case there is no doubt whatsoever that together these problems would affect his school performance and capabilities.

Although in the past it was felt to be a rare condition, Tourette syndrome is now recognized to be relatively common and most international studies show a prevalence of around 1 per cent of schoolchildren. There is a wide range of severity, so not all these cases would actually experience much difficulty in their schooling. It's interesting that in SEN settings the prevalence is somewhat higher. We have conducted several epidemiological studies in the UK and our published results concur with these figures. We have also calculated how many youngsters in this country may have Tourette syndrome and it is at least around 100 000. It is thus imperative that the educational services understand and are able to include youngsters with this problem in their educational strategy. Most, but not all, patients improve by the age of 18.

I am in no way suggesting that Johnny has an intellectual difficulty. I am also in no doubt whatsoever that Johnny has Tourette syndrome and it is unquestionably a medical disorder.

Some suggestions for strategies to help in the class and in examinations are as follows:

1. It is imperative to note that children cannot help the tics and in general penalizing children for this is unhelpful.

2. Sometimes youngsters with Tourette syndrome benefit from a little 'time out' of the classroom. This must be in no way punitive, but it can give a break from the classroom setting and if they're being noisy it may give the other youngsters a short break too.

3. Reading out questions to the child can lead to better comprehension than individual reading by the child.

4. I strongly suggest that Johnny be given more time in examinations, and he may well benefit from sitting the exam in a separate room with

an individual invigilator. I would not want Johnny to be singled out, but many of our youngsters find that this is particularly helpful as being in a classroom at times stresses them, and the stress of suppressing tics in public in an examination situation obviously leads to very unhelpful self-consciousness, especially when there is the possibility of disturbing other candidates.

5. Many youngsters with Tourette syndrome find that it is helpful to sit their examinations on a computer as this helps with many of the writing, timing, and other difficulties which are inherent in Tourette syndrome in the examination situation.

6. Some youngsters with Tourette syndrome necessitate a Statement of Special Educational Needs. In Johnny's case I would both suggest and support that.

7. Clearly, teasing and bullying needs to be addressed, a topic where the expertise lies entirely with you rather than me. There are very many examples of children with Tourette syndrome who have flourished in a supportive school atmosphere without experiencing significant teasing.

I have included a list of publications intended for lay and professional individuals in the communities besides doctors. In particular I would like to draw your attention to the book *Tourette Syndrome: A Practical Guide for Teachers, Parents and Carers*, by Amber Carroll and Mary Robertson, published by David Fulton, London, 2000. I do not suggest that you buy this book, although you may do so if you want to, but I certainly suggest that you obtain this from your local library as it is helpful and not only gives in much more detail what Tourette syndrome is but also highlights many strategies for dealing with youngsters with Tourette syndrome in the educational system, such as developing and valuing the individual, forming good relationships, focusing on positive behaviour, and ensuring that inclusion is a process and not a state. I have had good feedback from many teachers who have found the book extremely helpful not only for Tourette syndrome generally but also with particular youngsters with the disorder.

Tourettes Action can also be a valuable resource and further information is available at www.tourettes-action.org.uk. In fact, they can provide a booklet which also goes over some of this ground.

There can obviously be a very major impact on schooling. Indeed, the involuntary movements might not necessarily be the most disabling part of this; in many children they are merely a marker for some of the other problems that are going on underneath as described above.

With best wishes

Yours sincerely

Mary M Robertson MBChB, MD, DSc (Med), DPM, FRCP (UK), FRCPCH, FRCPsych

Emeritus Professor in Neuropsychiatry University College London

Visiting Professor & Hon Consultant St George's Hospital & Medical School

Hon Medical Advisor Tourettes Action

Index

TS = Tourette Syndrome

Abdul-Rau, Mahmoud 109
ablative structural surgery 81
ADHD *see* attention-deficit-
    hyperactivity disorder (ADHD)
adolescence 57
adult-onset tic disorder 32
affective disorders 41
age
    diagnosis 51
    increasing age, effect on
        symptoms of 44–6
    obsessive-compulsive behaviour, effect of
        increasing age on 45, 46
    onset of TS 16, 32, 43–4
    worst severity 45
alcohol 8
allergies 73
American DSM Classification 64
anger
    diagnosis 51, 53
    management 40
antibasal ganglia antibodies
    (ABGA) 27, 72
    antidepressants 54, 78
antipsychotics 77, 80
anxiety 39
anxiolytics 77
aripiprazole 78
assessments 22, 25–8, 63
associated features and disorders
    24–5, 28, 35–41, 76 *see also*
    attention-deficit-hyperactivity
    disorder (ADHD); obsessive–
    compulsive behaviour (OCB)
attention-deficit–hyperactivity disorder
    (ADHD) 12, 33–4
    assessments 26
    characteristics 24, 37
    clonidine 78
    diagnosis 28
    driving 105
    education 9, 84–7, 92, 100
    medication 6, 9, 78, 88
    prevalence 37, 41
    time outs 100
autistic spectrum disorders 18, 33,
    34, 85
autoimmune mechanisms 72
autosomal dominant inheritance 70
Aykroyd, Dan 109

bacterial infection 27
basal ganglia 27, 68–9, 72
behaviour therapies 76
Bennett, Pete 102, 109, 113–15
Bernotas, Eric 109
bibliography 129–41
birth factors 72–3
blame 53, 54–5
blinking 10, 16, 76
blood tests 27, 28–9, 63
Bonaparte, Napoleon 109
borderline personality disorder 40
brain scans 27, 68–9
bullying 7–8, 55–6, 87–8, 91

cannabis 8
caregiver burden 46, 56
case studies 3–12
causes of TS 67–73
    allergies 73
    biochemical causes 67–8

causes of TS (*cont.*)
  birth factors 72–3
  brain, affected areas of 68
  electrophysiology 68
  genetic factors 69–71
  hormones and stress 73
  infections 72
  neuroimaging 68–9
  psychology aetiology 72
celebrities 101–2, 107–26
Centanni, Louis 109
Change for Children programme 89
child psychologists 5–6
chocolate, caffeine or Coca Cola
    (the three Cs) 73
chromosomes 63, 71
chronic multiple motor or vocal tic
    disorder (CMTD) 32
clonidine 7
Cobain, Kurt 109
cognitive behavioural therapy (CBT) 13
Cohen, Brad 109
Collins, Keith 109
commencement of TS 16, 43–4
comorbid conditions 62, 69
compulsions *see* **obsessive–compulsive**
    behaviour (OCB)
computed tomography (CT) 27, 68–9
concentration, lack of 5, 7, 9, 37, 86
conduct disorder 34, 40, 87
contingency management 76
coping with diagnosis 49–59
coping with TS 57
coprographia (writing foul words) 126
coprolalia (inappropriate and
    involuntary swearing) 1, 6–7, 15, 23
  age 44
  diagnosis 19, 21, 64, 101
  education 84, 91
  Johnson, Samuel 113
  media 101
  mental coprolalia (thinking obscene
      thoughts) 15
  Mozart, WA 126
copropraxia (involuntary making
    of inappropriate obscene
    gestures) 15, 23, 84
copying behaviour 8
coughing 8

counselling 54, 57, 75
cures, searching for 53
cutting 24–5
cyclic-AMP 67–8

deep brain stimulation (DBS) 81
definition of TS 13–16
denial 50–1
Department for Children, Schools and
    Families 89–91
depression 25, 26, 34, 39, 54, 78, 79,
    87–8, 91, 113
development of other conditions 35–41
diagnosis
  age 51
  anger 51, 53
  assessments 22, 25–8
  associated features and disorders
      24–5, 28
  attention-deficit–hyperactivity
      disorder (ADHD) 28
  awareness 19–20
  blame 53
  blood tests 28–9, 63
  coping with diagnosis 49–59
  coprolalia 19, 21, 64, 101
  denial 50–1
  early diagnosis 21, 28–9
  emotional reactions 50–9
  guilt 49–50, 51, 54
  immediate consequences 58–9
  increased frequency of diagnoses 19–20
  late diagnosis 28–9
  making the diagnosis 21–9
  negligence 53
  over-diagnosis 20
  parents, reaction of 49–56
  phenotypes 63
  referrals 22
  relief 52
  shock 50–1, 58
  symptoms 22–5
  tests 19, 28–9, 63
  tics 22–3, 28–9
  unitary condition, TS as 62
diet 73
disability discrimination 92, 102, 104
distinguishing TS from other
    conditions 31–4

dopamine 52, 67–8, 71, 77, 79
Doran, Mort 92, 109, 115–17
double-blind trials 77
driving 105, 106
drugs *see* **medication**
DSM Classification 64
dyslexia 38–9
dyspraxia 38
dystonia 32, 80

'E' points 83–4
Early Years Action and Early Years Action Plus 96
echolalia (involuntary echoing back of speech of others) 1–2, 8, 15, 23, 33, 84, 113
echopraxia (imitation of other people's speech) 15, 23, 84
education 84–102, 106
    attention-deficit–hyperactivity disorder (ADHD) 9, 84–7, 92, 100
    autistic spectrum disorders 85
    behavioural difficulties 84–5
    bullying 87–8, 91
    case studies 4–9
    Change for Children programme 89
    communication 92
    concentration, lack of 86
    conduct disorder 87
    coprolalia 84, 91
    copropraxia 84
    decision-making, pupil involvement in 96
    Department for Children, Schools and Families 89–91
    depression 91
    disability discrimination 104
    doctors, role of 99–100, 157–60
    Early Years Action and Early Years Action Plus 96
    echolalia 84
    echopraxia 84
    faith schools 97–8
    further education institutes, types of 99
    goals that must be incorporated into education, basic 89–92
    grant-maintained schools 98
    Higher National Certificate (HNC) and Higher National Diploma (HND) 99

home tuition 98
homework 36, 86
independent schools 98
intelligence 86
leaflets, videos, and books 100
learning difficulties 84–5, 98
letters, doctors writing formal 99–100, 157–60
literature 100
mainstream schools 97–8
medication
    administration 97
    doctors, letters from 100
    side effects of 87–8
National Curriculum 88–92, 98, 101
National Healthy School Programme (NHSP) 91
National Vocational Qualification (NVQs) 99
neuropsychological problems 87
obsessive–compulsive behaviour (OCB) 36, 84–6
peers, effect on 85
personal, social and health education, curriculum for (PSHE) 91
personality disorder 87
Personalized Learning Strategy 89
portage (home based support for pre-school children) 98
problems at school, types of 85–8
public, educating the 84, 101–2
pupil referral units (PRUs) 98
rages and anger 90
relationships, forming 90–1
school phobia and school refusal 87–8
self-esteem and self-confidence 89, 90, 91, 100
self-injurious behaviour (SIB) 84
sixth form colleges 98
sources of information 89
special schools 98, 106
sport 100
stages of education system 98–9
Statements of Special Educational Needs 85, 92–6, 104
tics in schoolchildren, prevalence of 84–5, 88
time outs 100
transfer to different schools 89–90

education (*cont.*)
   TS associations and foundations 100
   TS, persons with 84–101
   types of school 97–8
   universities 99
   visuospatial deficits 86
   warning signs 90
   websites 101
Eisenreich, Jim 109, 117–18
electrocardiogram (ECG) 27
electroencephalogram (EEG) 27, 68
electrophysiology 68
emotional reactions to diagnosis 50–9
employment 102–3, 106
   disability discrimination 102, 104
   social security benefits 102–3
empowerment 103–5
environmental factors 45
epilepsy 27, 33, 56, 81
ethnic origins 18, 20
Evans, Richard Paul 109
executive dysfunction 38
expert witnesses 105–6
extreme reactions 53–4
eyes 5, 10, 16, 76

faith schools 97–8
families 45–6, 49–50, 52–3, 55–8, 76
family planning 57–8
famous or successful people with
   TS 101–2, 107–26
Faulkner, Noel 109
feedback forms and fact sheets 28, 153–6
fluoxetine 12, 78
food allergies 73
forms of TS 3
friends
   making 5, 8, 90–1
   talking about problems to 57–8
full-blown TS 62
functional brain studies 69
functional magnetic resonance imaging
   (fMRI) 27
further education institutes, types of 99

gender 20
genetic factors 12, 20, 46, 53–5, 57, 69–71
   autosomal dominant inheritance 70
   bilinear inheritance 70

   genotypes and phenotypes 63–4
   mixed model 70
   obsessive–compulsive behaviour
      (OCB) 36, 70
   polygenic model 70
genotypes 63, 64
gestures, making involuntary obscene
   (copropraxia) 15, 23, 84
government
   Department for Children, Schools and
      Families 89–91
   departments, guidelines and documents
      from 84
   early day motions 104–5
   information 84, 104–5
grant-maintained schools 98
group A beta-haemolytic
   streptococcus (GABHS) 72
guilt 49–50, 51, 54

habit reversal training 76
habits 4–12, 76, 117
Haines, Kellie 109, 118–19
haloperidol 79, 87, 117
heart problems 90
helpline 58
hereditary factors *see* genetic factors
Higher National Certificate (HNC)
   and Higher National
   Diploma (HND) 99
historical perspective of TS 62
holidays 58
Hollenbeck, Peter 92, 109, 119–20
home tuition 98
homework 36, 86
hormones and stress 73
Howard, Tim 92, 101–2, 109, 120–1
Huntington's disease 32, 63

ICD (WHO) criteria 64
imitation of other people's speech
   (echopraxia) 15, 23, 84
independent schools 98
infections 72
information, sources of 2–3, 19–20, 58,
   84, 89, 100, 103–5
international contacts and
   associations 143–52
Internet 101, 102–4

interview schedules 25
introductory cards 127
IQ testing 27
Itard, Jean Marc Gaspard 1, 44, 64

Johnson, Samuel 2, 109, 112–13
Johnston, Mike 109

leaflets 58, 100
learning difficulties 18, 33, 84–5, 98
    see also Statements of Special
    Educational Needs
letters to schools from doctors
    99–100, 157–60
literature 1–3, 19–20, 84, 100, 103

magnetic resonance imaging (MRI)
    27, 68–9
Malraux, André 109
mania 25
marriage or relationships,
    effect on 54–5
massed negative practices 76
McConnell, James 109
McKinley, Duncan 109, 122–3
media 101–2
medication 77–80
  age 97
  antidepressants 54, 78
  antipsychotics 77, 80
  anxiolytics 77
  aripiprazole 78
  attention-deficit–hyperactivity disorder
    (ADHD) 6, 9, 78, 88
  clonidine 78, 80, 87
  conduct disorder 40
  depression 54, 78, 79, 87–8
  doctors, letters to school from 100
  dopamine 67–8, 77, 79
  double-blind trials 77
  Eisenreich, Jim 117
  fluoxetine 12, 78
  haloperidol 79, 87, 117
  heart problems 80
  Hollenbeck, Peter 120
  list of common medications 79
  major tranquillizers 77
  management and administration 97
  methylphenidate 6, 7, 67, 78, 88

neuroleptics 32, 77–8, 79, 80
obsessive–compulsive
    behaviour (OCB) 78
oppositional defiant disorder 34, 39–40
pemoline 67
pimozide 79, 80, 87
risperidone 77, 87
schizophrenia 41
schools
  administration 97
  doctors, letters from 100
  side effects of 87–8
sedation 80
selective serotonin reuptake inhibitors
    (SSRIs) 78, 80
side effects 78, 79–80, 87–92, 98,
    101, 117
stimulants 78
sulpiride 77, 79, 87
tetrabenazine 80
tiapride 7
tics 41, 77–9
tranquillizers 77
trials 77
ziprasidone 77–8
memory deficits 38
mental coprolalia (thinking obscene
    thoughts) 15
mental palilalia (silently saying to
    oneself last part of word heard) 15
mental state examinations 25
methylphenidate (Concerta) 6, 7, 67,
    78, 88
Mihok, Dash 109
mimicking 8
Monk, Thelonius 110
motor (involuntary muscle movements)
    tics 1, 13–14, 18, 22–3, 28, 63
Mozart, Wolfgang Amadeus 126
MRI (magnetic resonance imaging)
    27, 68–9
multidisciplinary clinics 28
myoclonic epilepsy 33
myths 47, 65, 106, 126

Napoleon Bonaparte 109
National Curriculum 88–92, 98, 101
National Healthy School Programme
    (NHSP) 91

National Vocational Qualification (NVQs) 99
negligence in diagnosis 53
Nerdum, Odd 109, 123
neuroimaging 68–9
neuroleptics 32, 77–8, 79, 80
neurological examinations 25
neuropsychological problems 27, 38–9, 87
neurosurgery 80–1
neurotransmitters 67–8
noises 6–7, 8, 9
non-obscene socially inappropriate behaviours (NOSI) 24, 37–8

obsessive–compulsive behaviour (OCB) 9–10, 12, 33–4, 41
  age, effect of increasing 45, 46
  assessments 26
  behaviour therapy 76
  compulsions, examples of 24, 36
  Doran, Mort 116, 117
  education 36, 84–6
  genetic factors 36, 70
  infections 72
  Johnson, Samuel 112, 113
  medication 78
  obsessions, examples of 24, 36
  selective serotonin reuptake inhibitors (SSRIs) 78
  self-injury 36
  self-injurious behaviour (SIB) 37
  tics 36, 45, 46
obsessive–compulsive disorder (OCD) 69
OCB *see* obsessive–compulsive behaviour onset, age of 32, 43–6
oppositional defiant disorder 34, 39–40

paediatric autoimmune neuropsychiatric disorders associated with streptococcal infections (PANDAS) 72
palilalia (repetition of patient's own last words) 6, 15, 23
palipraxia (repetitive movements) 23
parents
  diagnosis, reaction to 49–56
  marriage or relationships, effect on 54–5

Statements of Special Educational Needs 96
  tics 52
Parkin, Luke 110
Parkinson's disease 81
peer-reviewed papers on the Internet 102–3
Peete, Calvin 110
pemoline 67
personal, social, and health education, curriculum for (PSHE) 91
personality disorders 34, 40, 41, 87
Peter the Great 109, 110–12
phenotypes 63–5
Picker, Tobias 110
pimozide 79, 80, 87
positive reinforcement 76
positron emission tomography (PET) 27, 69
prevalence of TS 2–3, 17–20, 46, 62
prognosis of TS 46
psychology aetiology 72
psychotherapy 76
public, educating the 84, 101–2
pupil referral units (PRUs) 98

quality of life (QoL) 45–6, 56

rages and angers 40, 90
rating scales 25
referral bias 41
relationships
  effect of TS on 54–5
  forming 5, 8, 90–1
relatives, talking about problems to 57–8
relaxation training 76
relief at diagnosis 52
remissions 46
repetition of patient's own last words (palilalia) 6, 15, 23
repetitive movements (palipraxia) 23
research 63–5, 71–2
risperidone 77, 87

Sacks, Oliver 92, 108, 119
samples, clinic versus community 41
Sandstrak, Pelle 109, 124–5
schizophrenia 25, 41, 52

schools 4–9
sedation 80
selective serotonin reuptake inhibitors
    (SSRIs) 78, 80
self-esteem and self-confidence 89, 90,
    91, 100
self-injurious behaviour (SIB) 24–5,
    36–7, 84
self-reporting 25–6
SENDS see Statements of Special
    Educational Needs 8
sensory integration dysfunction 38
serotonin 67–8
shock at diagnosis 50–1, 58
siblings 52–3, 55–7
side-effects of medication
    78, 79–80, 117
silently saying to oneself last part of
    word heard (palilalia) 15
simple TS 62
single-photon emission computed
    tomography (SPECT) 27, 69
sixth form colleges 98
Skaug, Joshua James William 110
Slattery, Ryan 110
sleep 4
SLITRK1 71
sniffing 10–11, 16
social security benefits 102–3
social skills deficit 38
spasmodic torticollis 32
special educational needs see
    Statements of Special
    Educational Needs
special schools 98, 106
specialists 11–12
SPECT (single-photon emission
    computed tomography) 27, 69
speech, imitation of other people's
    (echopraxia) 15, 23, 84
speech of others, echoing back of
    (echolalia) 1–2, 8, 15, 23, 33,
    84, 113
sport 8, 100
squinting 5, 10
SSRIs (selective serotonin reuptake
    inhibitors) 78, 80
St Vitus' dance 32
standard and self-reporting scales 25–6

Statements of Special Educational
    Needs 85, 92–7, 104
    Annual Reviews 96
    appeals 95
    codes of practice 96
    disability discrimination 92
    identification and assessment 93–4
    Individual Education Plans (IEP) 95
    Multi-Professional
        Assessments (MPAs) 95
    Notice in Lieu of a Statement 96
    OFSTED (Office for Standards in
        Education) 96
    parents and carers 96
    parts 94–5
    people involved in process 95–6
    pupil participation 96
    reports 92
    resource-led statementing 96
    School Action and School Action
        Plus 93–4
    special needs co-ordinators (SENCO) 95
    Transition Plan 96
    wave provision 93
Stenberg, Jeremy 'Twitch' 110
stereotypies 33
stigma 84, 88
stimulants 78
streptococcal infection 72
stress 73
structural brain studies 68–9
subtle neuropsychological
    deficits 38–9
successful people with TS
    101–2, 107–26
sulpiride 12, 77, 79, 87
surgery 80–1
swearing see coprolalia (inappropriate
    and involuntary swearing)
Swinburne, Algernon Charles 109
Sydenham's chorea
    (St Vitus' dance) 32
symptoms 3–12, 22–5, 64 see also tics

tardive dyskinesia 32, 79, 80
tardive tourettism 32
talking 4–5
teasing 55–6, 88, 119
telephone helpline 58

telling a child about their condition 56–7
temper tantrums 4, 6
tests 19, 27, 28–9, 63
tetrabenazine 80
therapies 75–81 *see also* **medication**
  associated disorders, persons with 76
  counselling 54, 57, 75
  neurosurgery 80–1
  types 76–81
thinking obscene thoughts (mental coprolalia) 15
throat, clearing of the 6, 7–8, 11–12, 16
tiapride 7
tics and twitches 6–11
  adult-onset tic disorder 32
  age 32, 43–6
    increasing age, effect of 44–5, 46
    onset, age of 16, 43–4
    severity, age of worst 45
  allergy 73
  behavioural difficulties 18
  birth, complications during 72
  bouts 45
  build-up 8
  chronic multiple motor or vocal tic disorder (CMTD) 32
  complex tics 1, 14, 15, 23
  control 14
  definition 13–14
  Doran, Mort 115–16
  Eisenreich, Jim 117
  environmental factors 45
  factors affecting tics 15–16
  functional brain studies 69
  habit reversal training 76
  Haines, Kellie 118
  head and face 22
  Hollenbeck, Peter 119
  infections 72
  Johnson, Samuel 113
  learning difficulties 18
  massed negative practices 76
  McKinley, Duncan 122
  medication 41, 77–9
  motor (involuntary muscle movements) tics 1, 13–14, 18, 22–3, 28, 63

  multidimensional tics 19
  obsessive–compulsive behaviour (OCB) 36, 45, 46
  parents' reaction 52
  peaking 45
  Peter the Great 111–12
  prevalence 18, 84–5, 88
  school children 84–5, 88
  shoulders 22–3
  simple motor tics 14, 23
  sport 100
  suppression 14, 88, 116
  tension 8, 14, 88
  transient tic disorder (TTD) 32
  twin studies 65
  urges 14
  vocal or phonic (noises) tics 1, 13–14, 22, 23, 28, 63
Tolstoy, Dmitry 109
Tolstoy, Leo 109
touching rituals 11, 16, 36, 117, 125
Tourette, Georges Gilles de la 1–2, 19, 62, 64
Tourettes Action 7, 11, 58, 71, 100, 102, 103, 106, 113–116, 152, 155, 159, 160
tranquillizers 77
transient tic disorder (TTD) 32
transport 104, 105
travel expenses, refunds and payment of 103
trials of medication 77
trisomy 21 63
TS plus 62
twin studies 65
twitches *see* **tics and twitches**
types of TS 61–5

under-achieving 20
unidentified TS 18, 20, 108
unitary condition, TS as 62, 64
universal prevalence of TS 20
universities 86

vocal or phonic (noises) tics 1, 13–14, 22, 23, 28, 63

Wallace, Steve 110
websites 101
Wechter, Julius 109
weight 4, 6, 27, 88
William of Orange 109
Wilson's disease 26, 33

Wolff, Michael 110
**words, writing foul
(coprographia)** 126

ziprasidone 77–8